Recipes on the Move in Early Modern England and British North America

Connected Histories in the Early Modern World

Connected Histories in the Early Modern World contributes to our growing understanding of the connectedness of the world during a period in history when an unprecedented number of people—Africans, Asians, Americans, and Europeans—made transoceanic or other long distance journeys. Inspired by Sanjay Subrahmanyam's innovative approach to early modern historical scholarship, it explores topics that highlight the cultural impact of the movement of people, animals, and objects at a global scale. The series editors welcome proposals for monographs and collections of essays in English from literary critics, art historians, and cultural historians that address the changes and cross-fertilizations of cultural practices of specific societies. General topics may concern, among other possibilities: cultural confluences, objects in motion, appropriations of material cultures, cross-cultural exoticization, transcultural identities, religious practices, translations and mistranslations, cultural impacts of trade, discourses of dislocation, globalism in literary/visual arts, and cultural histories of lesser studied regions (such as the Philippines, Macau, African societies).

Recipes on the Move in Early Modern England and British North America

Domestic Medicine, Mobility, and Manuscript Culture

Hillary M. Nunn

Amsterdam University Press

Cover illustration: Recipe for the coral tincture used in the "Great Cordial" recipe, Sandys Family Recipe Book, *English Receipt Book*, seventeenth century, Princeton MS RTC01 no. 208, Princeton University, 29r. Courtesy of Manuscripts Division, Department of Special Collections, Princeton University Library.

Cover design: Coördesign, Leiden
Lay-out: Crius Group, Hulshout

ISBN	978 94 6372 339 8
e-ISBN	978 90 4855 743 1 (pdf)
e-ISBN	978 90 4857 179 6 (accessible ePub)
DOI	10.5117/9789463723398
NUR	685

Table of Contents

List of Figures

Acknowledgments

It might seem fitting that a book about domestic medicine began to take shape during a pandemic lockdown. Discussions about health and mobility were in the air, and, thankfully, librarians and scholars alike were willing to offer input and support virtually to this project. Their contributions, along with the insights of those who helped to shape this project in person during its earlier stages and face-to-face in more recent months, made a substantial impact on this book.

I would like to thank Amsterdam University Press, with special gratitude to commissioning editor Erika Gaffney for her generous and kind help with the volume's preparation. Deep appreciation is due, as well, to series editor Julia Schleck and to those who offered peer review feedback, which made this volume stronger and more cohesive.

The University of Akron, especially the Faculty Research Committee, the Buchtel College of Arts and Sciences, and the Department of English, provided valuable financial support of this project. A Consortium for History of Science, Technology and Medicine Fellowship made much of the research possible, and meetings with its fellows provided valuable feedback during COVID shutdowns.

I am also grateful to the College of Physicians of Philadelphia, and to the Francis Clark Wood Institute, for facilitating my visits to their collections. Sarah Heim at the Kislak Center at the University of Pennsylvania and Alain St. Pierre at the Princeton University Firestone Library provided invaluable support in accessing the manuscripts at the core of this book. Without the generosity of librarians at the New York Academy of Medicine and the Virginia History Center, this book would never have been completed. I am particularly grateful to Kim Wilson May at the Museum of Early Southern Decorative Arts (MESDA) Research Center in Winston-Salem and Matthew Guillen at the Virginia Museum of History & Culture for providing virtual access to materials, and to Tom Richardson at the North Yorkshire County Record Office and Philip Bye at the East Sussex Records Office for their online consultation. The research in chapter 1 originally appeared in the *Journal for Early Modern Cultural Studies*, and I thank them for their efforts to see that work into print.

Conversations at the Folger Shakespeare Library brought this book into focus, and meetings at the Newberry Library helped underscore the breadth of recipe studies in the early modern period. Colleagues working with recipes and early modern science enriched this project greatly. I am forever grateful to Madeline Bassnett, Liza Blake, Michelle DiMeo, David Goldstein, Marissa Nicosia, Jennifer Park, Whitney Sperrazza, and Amy Tigner for their support, conversation, and feedback. Edith Snook's enormous generosity made revisions to early drafts much more productive. Mackie Black's attention to detail has benefited this project immensely as well. I owe particularly big thanks to Rebecca Laroche and Melissa Schultheis, who brought me into generative collaborative projects.

The Early Modern Recipes Online Collective provided a community that enabled this work in an area that has grown immensely in recent years. Steering committee members Elaine Leong, Jennifer Munroe, Margaret Simon, and Lisa Smith eagerly offered advice and feedback. Julia Nurse at the Wellcome Collection, and Gail Chapman and Pamela Forde at the Royal College of Physicians of London, as well as scores of student recipe transcribers, have helped reinforce my enthusiasm for working with manuscripts that have been so often overlooked. We all owe great thanks to Heather Wolfe at the Folger Shakespeare Library, whose devotion to collecting and transcribing recipe manuscripts has made this work possible.

Finally, I would like colleagues Alan Ambrisco, Janet Bean, Yvonne Bruce, Patrick Chura, and Julie Drew for their good advice and even better humor. This project has also made me grateful for the members of my family who have shared their recipes with me, first among them my amazingly resourceful mother, Jean Nunn. Above all, thanks to Richard Wisneski who gave invaluable support throughout all stages of this volume's production.

Introduction: Recipes on the Move

Abstract: This introduction provides a framework for considering how recipe manuscripts reflect the habits of movement developing among English recipe compilers—and within their families and English culture more broadly—during the early modern period. Establishing the book's focus on healthcare recipes, the chapter offers a summary of current scholarship on early modern manuscript recipe books while integrating background on the increasing availability of imported ingredients in early modern England. Challenges to long-established ideas of the English humoral body are laid out as well, emphasizing the impact of transatlantic travel and settler colonialism on healthcare practices on both sides of the Atlantic ocean. An outline of the book's chapters concludes the section.

Keywords: manuscripts; *Airs, Waters, Places*; humors; settler colonialism; travel; Indigenous sources

To examine recipes is to examine movement. Recipes at their core require that their users act upon raw materials to create preparations that better suit intended purposes, whether these purposes involve making medical cures, preserving fruit, or roasting cuts of meat. Recipes as written in the early modern period emphasized motion from their opening words, demanding that users "take" and "put" ingredients together, rather than starting with the distinct, precise list of items and amounts expected of the form today. In the era's manuscript recipe collections, moreover, the titles affixed to these instructions commonly emphasized the tasks to be taken up, inviting us to see the maker as she works "To pickell barberies" or "To make poppie water."[1] Such phrasing helps us see the kitchenworker as preparing for labor, then concocting the medicines and foods needed to keep the household thriving.

1 Constance Hall, *Receipt Book*, 1672, Folger MS V.a.20, Folger Shakespeare Library, Washington, DC, 7r, 37v; Kowalchuk offers a full transcription of Hall's manuscript, where these recipes appear. See Kristine Kowalchuk, *Preserving on Paper: Seventeenth-Century Englishwoman's Receipt Books* (Toronto: University of Toronto Press, 2017), 166, 210.

Nunn, Hillary M. *Recipes on the Move in Early Modern England and British North America: Domestic Medicine, Mobility, and Manuscript Culture.* Amsterdam: Amsterdam University Press, 2025.
DOI 10.5117/9789463723398_INTRO

Indeed, William Eamon defines a recipe as "a prescription for taking action," noting that the word *recipe* is the Latin imperative "take," where that action is often experimental.[2] Even when part of repeated household routines, a recipe's steps can bring about different results, based on the maker's abilities, the quality of ingredients, or the surrounding environmental factors like season, weather, or location; such variables mean that the enacting of a recipe can in fact lead to different outcomes, even if it directs its users toward a specific desired end. As Debapriya Sarkar notes, early modern recipes typically "assume knowledge on the reader's part of external conditions as well as their familiarity with the task," relying on the maker's discretion about how and when to follow the outlined procedures.[3] The recipe constitutes what Julia Rhinehart Lupton sees as "a kind of script," where the unit of action it orchestrates can unfold "in a number of different procedural systems, such as daily meal preparation, preserving and candying, cosmetics and hygiene, medicines, minor surgery, housekeeping, and banqueting."[4] The motion required to perform these scripts, moreover, can alter their makers' physical and mental states.[5] In short, these multipurpose texts guide users toward predetermined ends, whether used for the first or the fiftieth time, but there is no guarantee that all users will get to the same place.

But early modern recipes do more than direct the movements of their users. Recipes—and the manuscripts where they were recorded—moved in their own right, traveling from household to household and from generation to generation. This is the restlessness that Sara Pennell and Michelle DiMeo emphasize in noting that the Latin *recipere* "stresses the mobility of the information carried by the text."[6] This is especially true

2 William Eamon, *Science and the Secrets of Nature* (Princeton: Princeton University Press, 1994), 131. For more on the notion of recipes as "received forms," see Sara Pennell and Michelle DiMeo, "Introduction," in *Reading and Writing Recipe Books, 1500–1800*, eds. Sarah Pennell and Michelle DiMeo (Manchester: Manchester University Press, 2013), 10.

3 For Sarkar, recipes need to be performed to fulfill their practice of "futuristic knowledge"; see Debipriya Sarkar, *Possible Knowledge: The Literary Forms of Early Modern Science* (Philadelphia: University of Pennsylvania Press, 2023), 58–62, esp. 60.

4 Julia Reinhard Lupton, "Thinking with Things," *Postmedieval: A Journal of Medieval Cultural Studies* 3, no. 1 (2012): 66.

5 These processes can become engrained in the maker's body as well. For more on the bodily knowledge that stems from interaction with recipe instructions, see Katherine Walker, "Instinct and the Body of the Early Modern Cook," in *In the Kitchen: 1550–1800: Reading English Cooking at Home and Abroad*, eds. Madeline Bassnett and Hillary M. Nunn (Amsterdam: Amsterdam University Press, 2022), 71–78; and Rebecca Laroche, "Minding the Fire," in *In the Kitchen: 1550–1800: Reading English Cooking at Home and Abroad*, eds. Madeline Bassnett and Hillary M. Nunn (Amsterdam: Amsterdam University Press, 2022), 221–27.

6 Pennell and DiMeo, "Introduction," 10.

of the entries in household manuscript recipe collections, which brought together and kept handy bits of knowledge that a compiler acquired from her own experiences, as well as from her friends, her family, and her social networks.[7] These recipes often proudly carry indications of their origins in other places, ranging from a neighbor's kitchen to lands on the other side of an ocean. Women in particular, Catherine Field observes, "were authorized to practice, write, and exchange technical 'how-to' knowledge in the areas of both food and medicine, an exchange that often occurred through the text of the recipe book."[8] Sometimes recipes journeyed from place to place as scribbled instructions on loose sheets of paper, written down during a visit or delivered as part of a letter, before being added to the keeper's recipe book. Other times, compilers incorporated recipes in bulk, copying them from the collections kept by friends and relatives when they had the chance. During her time in Spain in 1650, for example, Lady Ann Fanshawe acquired several pages worth of perfume recipes, which she then sewed into her own manuscript.[9] The path these pages took to meet her larger recipe collection remains uncertain, but they are clearly aggregated from a place separate from the rest of her book. And other times, recipe manuscripts themselves traveled, moving to new homes with their first owners or, as is often the case, with younger family members charged with running new households. Fanshawe's manuscript exemplifies both these kinds of movement, accompanying her on her family's own journeys throughout England and in Europe, before becoming a gift to Ann's daughter Katherine Fanshawe in 1678.[10]

7 On social networks and knowledge transmission in recipe books, see Michelle DiMeo, "Authorship and Medical Networks," in *Reading and Writing Recipe Books, 1550–1800*, eds. Michelle DiMeo and Sara Pennell (Manchester: Manchester University Press, 2013), 25–46; Elaine Leong, *Recipes for Everyday Knowledge* (Chicago: University of Chicago Press, 2018), 19–45; Sara Pennell, "Perfecting Practice?: Women Manuscript Recipes and Knowledge in Early Modern England," in *Early Modern Women's Manuscript Writing: Selected Papers from the Trinity/Trent Colloquium*, eds. Victoria E. Burke and Jonathan Gibson (Basingstoke: Ashgate, 2004), 237–58; and Wendy Wall, *Recipes for Thought: Knowledge and Taste in the Early Modern Kitchen* (Philadelphia: University of Pennsylvania Press, 2015), 18–19. For more on recipe manuscripts as a mode of preserving traditions while incorporating new practices, see Kowalchuk, *Preserving on Paper*, 29.

8 Catherine Field, "'Many Hands Hands': Writing the Self in Early Modern Women's Recipe Books," *Genre and Women's Life Writing in Early Modern England*, eds. Michelle M. Dowd and Julie Eckerle (Aldershot: Ashgate, 2007), 52.

9 Ann Fanshawe, *Mrs. Fanshawes Book of Receipts*, 1678, Wellcome MS 7113, Wellcome Library, London, England, 91r–93v.

10 Katherine Fanshawe signs her name in the manuscript collection's opening pages, indicating it was "Given mee by my Mother March [the] 23. 1678." See Fanshawe, *Mrs. Fanshawe's Booke of Receipts*, 1678, Wellcome MS 7113, 2r.

Early modern recipe manuscript compilations—those collections of handwritten recipes consulted and expanded over years, and sometimes generations—offer particularly valuable glimpses of the movement involved in this accrual, evaluation, and implementation of household knowledge. Much of the growing body of scholarship surrounding these manuscripts focuses on how they reflect the practices of a given household, concentrating on domestic knowledge communicated through women's familial networks.[11] Manuscript recipe collections served as portable archives of family history, recording the medical knowledge gleaned over generations, and sometimes over centuries. It would be a mistake, however, to envision these collections as wielding influence only in the houses where they resided. Elaine Leong and Wendy Wall, along with Michelle DiMeo and Sara Pennell, have established that these texts should shape our understanding of how domestic expertise overlaps with the social and scientific life of the early modern period.[12] As more libraries have provided digital images of their collections, and as transcription work by the Early Modern Recipes Online Collective has made these texts increasingly accessible, these manuscripts have begun to claim their place in scholarly conversations regarding life writing, scientific knowledge, and notions of embodiment.[13] Most recently, these manuscripts have also begun to inspire scholarly discussions about early modern trade's impact on culinary practices, with scholars paying particular attention to the absorption of recipes—sometimes called receipts[14]—from foreign sources, and of ingredients originating outside England, into English foodways.[15]

11 Surviving manuscript collections certainly support this appealing narrative of women's ownership, but men were often involved in these domestic projects as well. Pennell finds that recipe books attributed to women often reveal evidence of male scribal penmanship, and some men actively added to their families' medical handbooks. See Pennell, "Perfecting Practice?," 240–43. Elaine Leong argues that recipes books were commonly family projects, ones that involved the men of the house as well as the women. See Leong, *Recipes for Everyday Knowledge*, 23–27.

12 See Michelle DiMeo and Sara Pennell, eds., *Reading and Writing Recipe Books, 1500–1800* (Manchester: Manchester University Press, 2013); Leong, *Recipes for Everyday Knowledge*; and Wall, *Recipes for Thought*.

13 For more on the efforts of the Early Modern Recipes Online Collective, see Rebecca Laroche et al., "Becoming Visible: Recipes in the Making," *Early Modern Women* 13, no. 1 (2018): 133–43. The Manuscript Cookbooks Survey has been a valuable resource since 2011 for locating these manuscripts. See Stephen Schmidt and Szilvia Szmuk-Tanenbaum, "Manuscript Cookbooks Survey," Project of the Pine Needles Foundation of New York.

14 Wall suggests that the word *receipt* was more often used in relation to foods. See Wall, *Recipes for Thought*, 4. Given my focus on medical preparations, this book will chiefly use the term *recipe*.

15 For particularly vivid case studies, see Rob Wakeman, "The Power of the Pot: Naturalizing Carp Through the Early Modern English Receipt Book," in *In the Kitchen: 1550–1800: Reading English Cooking at Home and Abroad*, eds. Madeline Bassnett and Hillary M. Nunn (Amsterdam:

Traveling medical recipes in household manuscripts, on the other hand, have enjoyed less scholarly attention. These seemingly homely texts carried with them the potential to change domestic healthcare, transferring knowledge to new makers in different environments. Such recipes not only show us what afflictions household members wanted to tackle, but what materials and methods they could harness in those efforts. This study situates the household medical practices reflected in manuscript recipe collections within the era's expanding travel and trade networks, illuminating the connections between these domestic texts and the commercial world. As Londa Schiebinger argues in *Plants and Empire: Colonial Bioprospecting in the Atlantic World*, the drive to introduce American plants to the European market spurred ocean voyages and transformed eighteenth-century science.[16] Patrick Wallis's and Harold J. Cook's work shows that the arrival of these plants on English shores in the previous century had already begun to reshape medical practices, even in domestic situations, and Matthew James Crawford and Joseph M. Gabriel's collection *Drugs on the Page* traces the effect these imports had throughout Europe on the pharmacopeias designed to offer guidance to professional medical practitioners.[17] In England, the introduction of tobacco famously brought tremendous changes not just to social and economic life, but to healthcare as well. While its leisure use encouraged investment in the Virginia Company, the plant soon found its way into medical recipes, both in print and manuscript, where it treated wounds, miscarriage, and even breathing difficulties.[18]

Amsterdam University Press, 2022), 131–47 and Amy L. Tigner, "Cake: An Early Modern Chronicle of Trade, Technology, and Exchange," in *In the Kitchen: 1550–1800: Reading English Cooking at Home and Abroad*, eds. Madeline Bassnett and Hillary M. Nunn (Amsterdam: Amsterdam University Press, 2022), 109–27. For consideration of the impact of trade and travel on early modern culinary manuscripts in the Europe more broadly, see Sarah Peters Kernan and Helga Müllneritsch, eds., *Culinary Texts in Context, 1500–1800: Manuscript Recipe Books in Early Modern Europe* (Amsterdam: Amsterdam University Press, 2024).

16 See Londa Schiebinger, *Plants and Empire: Colonial Bioprospecting in the Atlantic World* (Boston: Harvard University Press, 2007).

17 See Harold J. Cook, "Markets and Cultures: Medical Specifics and the Reconfiguration of the Body in Early Modern Europe," *Transactions of the Royal Historical Society* 21 (2011): 123–45; Patrick Wallis, "Exotic Drugs and English Medicine: England's Drug Trade, c. 1550–1800," *Social History of Medicine* 25, no. 1 (2012): 20–46; and Matthew James Crawford and Joseph M. Gabriel, eds., *Drugs on the Page: Pharmacopoeias and Healing Knowledge in the Early Modern Atlantic World* (Pittsburgh: University of Pittsburgh Press, 2019).

18 For a concise consideration of tobacco in healthcare recipes, see Misha Ewen, *The Virginia Venture: American Colonization and English Society, 1580–1660* (Philadelphia: University of Pennsylvania Press, 2022), 126; Edward McLean Test addresses the plant's curative powers in *Sacred Seeds: New World Plants in Early Modern English Literature* (Lincoln: University of Nebraska

The attention scholars have lavished upon tobacco has begun to spread to other imports as well. Jennifer Park and Edward McLean Test, among others, have examined the impact of imported mumia and guaiacum, and such studies have continued to help situate English household medicine within the context of colonialism and global expansion.[19] My work adds sassafras to these focused discussions, building upon studies of the plant from Wallis, Russell Magnaghi, and Katrina Maydom for my discussion of early modern domestic rheumatism treatments.[20]

This book considers how the movement of medicinal recipes, particularly as recorded in manuscripts, influenced domestic healthcare in early modern English culture, in England and in the Atlantic world; in doing so, the pages that follow concentrate on manuscript recipes whose travels can be traced from one location to another. Some of these journeys are relatively short, involving carriage rides from the countryside to London, while others involve longer voyages to the Americas, particularly Jamestown and the colonies that came to surround it. The movement of people and goods involved in smaller scale expeditions often goes unnoticed, but these journeys create alliances and force connections just as transatlantic travels can. In fact, this book's later chapters underscore how movement among settlers in America brought changes to received medical practices, as recipes journeyed to different locations in the colonies and even traveled back to England. Recipe manuscripts like the one kept by the Saffin-Ellis family, for example, reflect years spent in America before moving eastward to England with their owners;[21] William Penn's son, meanwhile, prepared a copy of a

Press, 2019), 73–82. Lauren Working sees English tobacco habits as a tool for creating distinctions between themselves and the Indigenous they sought to dominate; see her "Tobacco and the Social Life of Conquest in London, 1580–1625," *The Historical Journal* 65 (2022): 30–48. Michael Ziser, meanwhile, offers an extended consideration of scholarly interest in tobacco's cultural impact on England; see Ziser, "Sovereign Remedies: Natural Authority and the *Counterblaste to Tobacco*," *William and Mary Quarterly* 62, no. 4 (2005): 719–44. Key among the works foregrounding that interest is Marcy Norton, *Sacred Gifts, Profane Pleasures: A History of Tobacco and Chocolate in the Atlantic World* (Ithaca: Cornell University Press, 2008).

19 On guaiacum, see Test, *Sacred Seeds: New World Plants in Early Modern English Literature*, 108–11; on mumia, see Jennifer Park, "Discandying Cleopatra: Preserving Cleopatra's Infinite Variety in Shakespeare's *Antony and Cleopatra*," *Studies in Philology* 113, no. 3 (2016): 595–633.

20 Russell M. Magnaghi, "Sassafras and its Role in Early American, 1562–1662," *Terra Incognita* 29, no. 1 (1997): 10–21. Maydom offers valuable tables showing trends in sassafras imports; see Katrina Elizabeth Maydom, "New World Drugs in England's Early Empire," PhD diss., (Cambridge University, 2018).

21 Several such traveling manuscripts are examined in chapter 5 of this volume. See, in addition, *Saffin-Ellis Miscellany*, 1716–62, University of Pennsylvania Ms. Codex 230, University of Pennsylvania, Philadelphia, PA.

recipe manuscript kept by his mother, Gulielma Maria Springett, to take to Pennsylvania which somehow never made the journey.[22] One manuscript, begun by Anna Cromwell in England but eventually making its way to Massachusetts and catalogued as part of Charles Brigham's account book, has folded within it an enigmatic note that the collection was "given to Sarah Sartell when she moved to Grafton amongst the Indians"; especially in its later pages, the collection incorporates many common American ingredients like sassafras and tobacco, suggesting that recipe keepers were gathering materials from trade with their fellow colonists and Indigenous tribes, as well as from overseas.[23]

Entangled Bodies, Traveling Recipes: Humoral Bodies and Settler Colonialism

Whether owners took their manuscript compilations along as they made seasonal journeys between country estates and city townhouses, or whether they carried recipes with them to colonial homesteads and shared them with new neighbors there, these manuscripts linked their compilers to ancestral homes as they learned to cope with, and use, the unfamiliar resources afforded by their new environments. At the same time, these domestic collections incorporated newly encountered recipes, copying them as distinct additions or using them to revise practices already written on manuscript pages. Blending new and old recipes as they moved, these moving manuscripts illustrate the ways that freshly acquired knowledge and forms of practice interact with established methods, often becoming indistinguishable in the process. For many historians of science, the importance of this mobility is core to knowledge-making, to the extent that Pamela Smith concludes that that knowledge itself "is now understood to be constituted

22 Evelyn Abraham Benson, *Penn Family Recipes: Cooking Recipes of William Penn's Wife, Gulielma* (York, PA: George Shumway, 1966), 1–2.

23 Charles Brigham, *Account Book [manuscript]*, 1650–1730, American Antiquarian Society Mss. Folios Vols. B, American Antiquarian Society, Worcester, MA, n.p. Select recipes using sassafras and tobacco appear on pages 163, 77, and 98. Determining which recipes were recorded in England but reflect trade with America, and which were recorded in America reflecting local ingredients, requires a far larger study. The manuscript is the subject of a thesis by Lori Lyn Price, "Gender and Domestic Medicine: Analysis of a Seventeenth-Century Receipt Book" (Master's thesis, Harvard Extension School, 2016); it has also earned attention in Rebecca J. Tannenbaum, *The Healer's Calling: Women and Medicine in Early New England* (Ithaca: Cornell University Press, 2002), 17–27 and Amanda Herbert, *Female Alliances: Gender, Identity, and Friendship in Early Modern Britain* (New Haven: Yale University Press, 2014), 110.

in part by movement." In the case of medical cures, movement affected the perceived qualities of materials, because people in different locations adapted them differently into local practice and because symptoms and diseases themselves met with different interpretations when they arrived in new places, resulting in new treatments. Such changes, all occurring as knowledge moved from place to place, leads Smith to conclude that "the routes that materials, practices, and knowledge take can be more important than their roots or originary forms."[24]

Smith's observation is a relief to anyone who has ever hoped to determine where the recipes in early modern household manuscripts originated. While these manuscripts sometimes gesture to a recipe's past—noting the name of the person who supplied it to the compiler, the locations where particular ingredients might be found, or even the manuscript or print source from which the recipe was taken—their deeper roots typically remain unclear.[25] Recipe texts nevertheless reveal patterns of recipe migration. As these recipes shift from place to place—often alongside the manuscript compilers who acquired, modified, and offered them to their own friends and relatives—they accumulate additional meanings. Travel across different regions shapes these recipes, altering their meanings even when their words remain somewhat stable. Recipes with no comments or emendations within a collection might be simply overlooked by users, falling out of favor or proving unnecessary in new locales. Other recipes, meanwhile, are refined to better suit their new locations or tempered to emphasize connections to the people who earlier used them. These manuscript recipes, in short, bring with them traces of the lands and waters they traverse, and they continue to accumulate such traces in each location they call home, even when those homes may prove only temporary.

While medical recipes could be detached from the people and places that initially produced them, the characteristics of the locations that nurtured their development still matter, and compilers often made note of these places when incorporating cures into their own manuscript collections. As easily as recipes might travel, they reflected the interactions between their environments and the people who lived in them. In country, urban,

24 Pamela H. Smith, "Nodes of Convergence, Material Complexes, and Entangled Itineraries," in *Entangled Itineraries: Materials, Practices, and Knowledge across Eurasia*, ed. Pamela H. Smith (Pittsburgh: University of Pittsburgh Press, 2019), 5.

25 This is particularly true of recipe manuscripts traced to compilers situated outside elite social circles. For a compelling exploration of social networks in these less documented classes, see Kimberley G. Connor, "Seeking Margaret Baker: Identifying the Author of Three Manuscript Receipt Books," *ABO: Interactive Journal for Women in the Arts, 1640–1830* 12, no. 1 (2022): 1–29.

and even colonial settings, healthcare remained a domestic duty overseen and administered by women, both in England and in its American colonies. Household cures were always the first, and often the only, treatments available for most conditions; most of these cures were made at home, often from readily available plants and animal products.[26] A household's surroundings thus contributed many of the raw materials used in medical care, creating a strong link between the patient's body and the particulars of the nonhuman world immediately surrounding it. In Jennifer Munroe's words, preparing a recipe in this (or indeed any) atmosphere involved a "range of activities and agents beyond the human" because the act of making it "depends on, even as it may aim to intervene in, seasonality, climatic conditions of sunshine, rain (or drought), and time, all of which must be observed, more than harnessed, by the person doing the gathering."[27] For Munroe, the resulting entwining of human and nonhuman exemplifies what Stacy Alaimo calls the "trans-corporal," where humans and the individual creatures, plants, and materials of the surrounding environment are entangled with one another, creating a larger, living network of interdependence. These interactions form the foundation of most recipes, which recorded for later consultation the actions that created particular remedies from specific local ingredients. While the recipe could be made in another place, its results would inevitably vary, even with the slightest shift of environmental factors.

Early modern recipe makers and healthcare authorities articulated this connection through their adherence to the notion that individual bodies developed in conjunction with the environments where they were born and reared. This notion—one that Alison Bashford and Sarah W. Tracy note as stressing human dependence on the environment rather than interdependence[28]—found its roots in the Hippocratic treatise *Airs,*

26 For an overview of English women's roles in medical care during the period, see Elaine Leong, "Collecting Knowledge for the Family: Recipes, Gender, and Practical Knowledge in the Early Modern English Household," *Centaurus* 55 (2013): 81–103; Anne Stobart, *Household Medicine in Seventeenth-Century England* (London: Bloomsbury, 2016); and Mary E. Fissell, "Women, Health, and Healing in Early Modern Europe," *Bulletin of the History of Medicine* 82, no. 1 (2008): 1–17. For particularly helpful case study, devoted to Grace Mildmay's healthcare activities, see Linda Pollock, *With Faith and Physic: The Life of a Tudor Gentlewoman, Lady Grace Mildmay, 1552–1620* (New York: St. Martin's, 1995). For a valuable treatment of English women's healthcare practices in the early years of the American colonies, see Tannenbaum, *The Healer's Calling.*

27 Jennifer Munroe, "Sympoeisis and Early Modern Cooking: Troubling the Boundaries of Human/Nonhuman," in *In the Kitchen: 1550–1800: Reading English Cooking at Home and Abroad*, eds. Madeline Bassnett and Hillary M. Nunn (Amsterdam: Amsterdam University Press, 2022), 34–35.

28 Alison Bashford and Sarah W. Tracy, "Introduction: Modern Airs, Waters, and Places," *Bulletin of the History of Medicine* 86, no. 4 (2012): 496.

Waters, Places (which, ironically, had traveled far from its own origins in ancient Greece). This treatise depicts human bodies as embedded in their surroundings, insisting that, in Charles E. Rosenberg's words, "Particular configurations of soils and wind, season and climate produce particular patterns of morbidity and mortality, temperament and physique."[29] It followed from these principles that humans should eat and drink what was native to their first surroundings to maintain optimal health. Indeed, it suggested that journeying too far from one's birthplace could be dangerous, and that "Home represented the best place to be healthy; it was where one's body had been shaped, and so was the place best fitted to its constitution."[30] These ideals magnified the power of domestic medicine, reinforcing the conviction that the cures made at home best addressed the suffering of its occupants. Presumably, those who shared the same humoral makeup would know the best treatments for their kin and could customize medical care for bodies they were uniquely qualified to understand. In addition, caregivers had to consider their patients' geographical origins to determine appropriate treatment, and the constitutions of those who were treated in places far from their homes would be less familiar to available practitioners.

While this fear of negative health consequences discouraged many from journeying from home, the *Airs, Waters, Places* tradition offered comfort to English travelers even as it caused trepidation. If all environments were built on an entanglement of human and nonhuman elements, then survival depended largely on understanding that balance, even in seemingly inhospitable spaces. Place, after all, held sway not just over human bodies; it governed the qualities of the living things and diseases that thrived there. Such logic offered comfort to English colonists in North America, where, in Joyce Chaplin's words, "each climate contained complexes of natural phenomena (both diseases *and* plants) peculiar to it."[31] The surroundings that produced the plants and animal materials that proved key to medical treatments endowed these cures with unique qualities that could not be duplicated in other locales, just as the diseases these cures treated did not surface in other places. While the diseases encountered across the Atlantic may have been unfamiliar to them, English settlers could remain confident that the plants found in those strange lands would provide appropriate cures. The idea that these cures

29 Charles E. Rosenberg, "Epilogue: *Airs, Waters, Places*. A Status Report," *Bulletin of the History of Medicine* 86, no. 4 (2012): 662.

30 Andrew Wear, "Place, Health, and Disease: The *Airs, Waters, Places* Tradition in Early Modern England and North America," *Journal of Medieval and Early Modern Studies* 38, no. 3 (2008): 450.

31 Joyce E. Chaplin, *Subject Matter: Technology, the Body, and Science on the Anglo-American Frontier, 1500–1676* (Cambridge, MA: Harvard University Press, 2013), 194.

sometimes worked as well in England—even though they were displaced from their native soil and sometimes used for diseases unknown beyond the Americas—forced practitioners to confront the notion that bodies native to both sides of the ocean might be more similar than distinct.[32]

When compilers moved to the Americas, the processes of settler colonialism governed the domestic realms they occupied, creating tensions between their previous attachments to natal lands and their new situations across the sea. The English mission, after all, was not solely to extract materials from the Americas, or to exploit its Indigenous peoples for economic gain, though such practices did occur. As Patrick Wolfe stresses, "The primary object of settler-colonization is the land itself" where the "dominant feature is not exploitation [of Indigenous people] but [their] replacement."[33] Like all settler colonialists, the English sought to stake a claim to the lands of the so-called New World. Settler colonialism aimed to change the land itself into a place that resembled home, in all respects, including the humoral. As Laurence Veracini explains, "Triumphant settler colonialism is, after all, a violent act against geography: settler colonialism turns someone else's place into space and then into place again. The latter place looks like the one the settlers left behind, or should."[34] These expectations placed tremendous pressure on settler household practices—practices that, in Kathryn Kish Sklar's words, seek "to reproduce daily life" in hopes not just of establishing roots for English ways in the Americas but of spreading their influence.[35] Amy Kaplan calls this mission "manifest domesticity," where "the conditions of domesticity often become markers that distinguish civilization from savagery."[36] Though Kaplan's work concentrates on nineteenth-century domestic texts, her sense that households nurtured "internal unity while impelling the nation outward to encompass the globe" applies just as easily to early English settlement in the Americas.[37]

32 Chaplin, *Subject Matter,* 172 and Martha K. Robinson, "New Worlds, New Medicines: Indian Remedies and English Medicine in Early America," *Early American Studies: An Interdisciplinary Journal* 3, no. 1 (2005): 99–100.

33 Patrick Wolfe, *Settler Colonialism and the Transformation of Anthropology: The Politics and Poetics of an Ethnological Event* (London: Cassell, 1999), 163.

34 Lorenzo Veracini, "Introduction: Settler Colonialism as a Distinct Mode of Domination," in *The Routledge Handbook of the History of Settler Colonialism*, eds. Edward Cavanagh and Lorenzo Veracini (New York: Routledge, 2016), 5.

35 Kathryn Kish Sklar, "Reconsidering Domesticity through the Lens of Empire and Settler Society in North America," *American Historical Review* 124, no. 4 (2019): 1250.

36 Amy Kaplan, "Manifest Domesticity," *American Literature* 70, no. 3 (1998): 582.

37 Kaplan, "Manifest Domesticity," 587. Sklar notes that settler colonialism's attention to domestic practices "also facilitated the analysis of domestic life as sites of conflict between

The logic of settler colonialism held that the English could change Virginia into a new homeland where they could thrive; long-standing principles of *Airs, Waters, Places*, meanwhile, proclaimed that the colonists should have simply stayed home. Indeed, it was English bodies that transformed, not the land, when they arrived in Virginia, just as Hippocratic medical traditions foresaw. What proved less predictable, however, was the English willingness to embrace these changes as a mark of this very same triumphant settler colonialism. Settlers, it turns out, understood that they needed to adapt to thrive in the climate now surrounding them. These processes of adjustment, often taking shape as a period of fever-filled illness vividly labeled *seasoning*, marked a perceived transformation within an English person's body. Survivors of this process—to be further discussed in chapter 4—could be assured of an earned harmony between themselves and their new environment, but at a cost. Even as the English insisted upon the differences between themselves and the Indigenous peoples of North America, settlers realized they needed to follow Algonquian ways for survival; these realizations, in turn, exerted profound strain upon English notions of their own biological identity. The English, that is, recognized that they could only survive in America by learning from Indigenous entanglements with their surroundings, even if this meant loosening the humoral connection that settlers envisioned as maintaining ancestral ties to their homelands.

The relief of surviving the physical adjustments of seasoning thus brought with it anxiety about identity and, though not fully articulated until the eighteenth century, race. As Suman Seth points out, increasing global movement raised questions about long-held convictions of the environment's responsibility for differences in human constitutions and complexions. As Seth puts it, "The idea of seasoning served as a solution to a problem concerning the ways that bodies changed as they entered new environments"; at the same time, English sufferers came through the illness without drastic changes to their appearance, challenging European ideas that "various racial features, such as skin colour or physiognomy" marked the bearer as belonging to their physical environment.[38] The physical impact of moving to a new land challenged English notions of their steadfast physical constitution, but those alterations in identity were more subtle than expected. The boundaries between themselves and the Indigenous were thus less

white settlers and Native people," using examples from the nineteenth and twentieth centuries. See Sklar, "Reconsidering Domesticity," 1256.

38 Suman Seth, "Race, Seasoning, and Strangeness: The Problem of Mobility in Early Modern Science and Medicine," *Global Intellectual History* 8, no. 4 (2022): 450.

clearly demarcated than the English had envisioned. Both reassuring and unsettling, the bodily changes that settlers experienced nonetheless left them in a kind of humoral limbo.

While such disruptions accompanied even small moves within England, the shock of a transatlantic crossing suggested a more drastic dislocation from English humoral identity. As Jean Feerick points out, the Virginia Company initially called upon this distance as a benefit, reframing the health challenges of colonization as purifying experiences that would strip away the corruptions of increasingly urban English life. But, she points out, "fears of degeneration lingered in the margins."[39] Such fears permeated the ranks of Spanish conquistadors, too, who shared with the English the notion that Indigenous foods would contaminate their bodies, subjecting them to a creeping Americanness. Not only would this attach them to a new environment; it would ruin the physical distinctions that determined their social status in Europe. As Rebecca Earle points out, conquistadors yearned to protect a *limpieza de sangre*, or purity of blood, demonstrated in Spain through a complicated blending of genealogy and reputation.[40] For the English, blood mattered in a more substantial, more grounded, way, one that reverberated with the logic of *Airs, Waters, Places*. In England, Feerick argues, "land was at the centre of this symbolics of blood, as we can observe in and through the period's naming practices whereby the nobility were named for the land that anchored their identity."[41] Individuals, that is, owed their sense of self to the place that they lived, especially if they had a family claim to that land. Moving across the ocean stretched, if not severed, that connection, creating a gap where new definitions of self might take root. The sense of displacement that came with English settler colonial efforts thus created an instability that, in Feerick's words, "catalys[ed] profound revaluations of the period's dominant account of blood. Efforts to reproduce the social body of England in new soils, that is, had the effect of unsettling the system of race then dominantly constituting England's social structure."[42] This instability, together with lingering anxieties regarding the environment's unsuitability for their constitutions, left English settlers fundamentally unsure of their physical attachment to either the so-called New or Old Worlds.

39 Jean Feerick, *Strangers in Blood: Relocating Race in the Renaissance* (Toronto: University of Toronto Press, 2010), 109.

40 Rebecca Earle, *The Body of the Conquistador: Food, Race and the Colonial Experience in Spanish America, 1492–1700* (Cambridge: Cambridge University Press, 2012).

41 Feerick, *Strangers in Blood*, 15.

42 Feerick, *Strangers in Blood*, 18.

The vast majority of manuscript transcribers featured in this book descended from what was considered noble blood, and in America fears of lost English identity threatened to overshadow brighter thoughts of new beginnings. Jane Bolling Randolph, however, embodies one small possibility of a counternarrative to worries stemming from the stress of dislocation with her claimed relationship to Pocahontas, famed daughter of Powhatan chief Wahunsenaca. Also known by the name Matoaka, Pocahontas had been celebrated in English accounts of Jamestown's founding as the savior of John Smith, and was popularly labeled American royalty.[43] According to nineteenth-century letters, Randolph's mother, born Jane Rolfe Bolling, was Pocahontas's granddaughter, and several family members recount the recipe compiler's father, John Bolling, as working to secure ownership of a portrait of Pocahontas that became a long-noted feature in the family home.[44] Forty years after Jane Randolph penned her recipe manuscript, a Bolling relative treated a journal-keeping visitor to enough genealogical detail that he could recount that Matoaka "left an only son, who was married, and left only daughters; those daughters, others; and thus it is, through the family line, that the blood of the fair Pocahontas now flows in the veins of the young and fair Mrs. Bolling."[45] This pride makes it all the more striking that Randolph's recipe manuscript offers little recognition of Algonquian influence in either medical or cookery recipes. Indeed, as Kevin Noble Maillard points out of Matoaka and similarly invoked Indigenous "princess" forebears today, "Pocahontas and her Grandmotherly counterparts exist as historical figures rather than present identities. Safely ensconced in a distant racial past, racial impurity normally inherited from non-White blood disappears."[46] As we shall see, however, traces of Indigenous knowledge in recipe practices linger in unacknowledged form.

43 For a useful summary of the English and Algonquian retellings of Pocahontas's life, see Lauren Working, "Pocahontas (c.1595–1617)," in *Lives in Transit in Early Modern England: Identity and Belonging*, ed. Nandini Das (Amsterdam: Amsterdam University Press, 2022), 185–92.

44 These family letters are quoted in Thomas Loraine McKenney and James Hall, *The Indian Tribes of North America with Biographical Sketches and Anecdotes of the Principal Chiefs* (Edinburgh: John Grant, 1934), 3: ix–xii.

45 Marquis de Chastellux, *Travels in North America in the Years 1780, 1781, and 1782*, trans. Howard C. Rice, Jr. (Chapel Hill: University of North Carolina Press, 1963), 2:424. The Marquis de Chastellux includes a three-page account of the Pocahontas myth before coming to this conclusion, 2:422–24.

46 Kevin Noble Maillard, "The Pocahontas Exception: The Exemption of American Indian Ancestry from Racial Purity Law," *Michigan Journal of Race & Law* 12, no. 2 (2007): 382. Maillard's study offers a fascinating reading of how Indigenous blood came to be seen as white within the Virginia legal system in the twentieth century, despite the state's interest in policing interracial

Recipe manuscripts reveal, in Jennifer Park's words, this "problem of cultural erasure and appropriation" in such omissions,[47] shifting origin stories to obscure the knowledge of Indigenous and enslaved peoples. This practice, as Londa Schiebinger sees it, indicates a pluralistic "Atlantic World medical complex," where Indigenous and European knowledges mix together, though more recently scholars have explicitly articulated this as European failure to acknowledge debts to their colonized counterparts.[48] Manuscripts that never left English soil reflect this bias whenever they record a recipe using tobacco or, as we shall see, sassafras without referencing American origins. Even when manuscripts recount the stories of a recipe's arrival from a non-English source, they often omit the names of those providing the cure. Amy L. Tigner describes, for instance, a cure for kidney stones in the Granville family manuscript, which focuses on the story of a Captain Thomas Phelps who "lerned & procured" a cure "from the moors" before passing the recipe to John Westcombe. "The moors" are the acknowledged source, but Westcombe, a family friend, serves as the named, local authority.[49]

This reliance upon—and temptation to obscure—the knowledge of Indigenous and enslaved peoples proves even more prevalent in English recipe manuscripts that established new roots in America. The lengthy communication trail involved in the transmission of this local knowledge from Indigenous sources to settlers was itself a contributor to such omissions, but, as Alisha Rankin argues, translators and intermediaries often purposely blurred recipe origins. Even when these European texts manage to offer glimpses of Indigenous healers at work—thus turning the text into an "archive of practice"—economic and cultural anxieties and,

marriage. "For elite Virginians to demand this accommodation demonstrates a malleable and shifting concept of racial purity. In conceptualizing the damning influence and palpable threat of 'taint' to White racial identity, strains of Indian blood assume a different, more exotic and arguably desirable meaning," Maillard writes before concluding, "At the same time, no adjustments existed to protect Black ancestry." See Maillard, "The Pocahontas Exception," 355.

47 Jennifer Park, "Teaching Recipes, Race, and Erasure in the Early Modern Classroom," *Studies in Medieval and Renaissance Teaching* 28, no. 2 (2021): 61–79.

48 Londa Schiebinger, *Secret Cures of Slaves: People, Plants, and Medicine in the Eighteenth-Century Atlantic World* (Stanford: Stanford University Press, 2017), 3; for a valuable account of the ways that circulation of medical knowledge within non-European communities in the Americas influence the archive of practice, see Pablo F. Gómez, "[Un]Muffled Histories: Translating Bodily Practices in the Early Modern Caribbean," *Osiris* 37 (2022): 233–50.

49 Amy L. Tigner, "Trans-border Kitchens: Iberian Recipes in Seventeenth-Century English Manuscripts," *History of Retailing and Consumption* 5, no. 1 (2019): 57–59. The recipe appears in Granville Family, *Cookery and Medical Receipts of the Granville Family, c. 1640–c. 1750*, Folger MS V.a. 430, Folger Shakespeare Library, Washington, DC, 122 and is transcribed in Kowalchuk, *Preserving on Paper*, 110.

most significantly, worries about authority obscured these accounts.[50] For example, Jane Randolph calls for "half an oz: of Kipscacuanna" in her manuscript's "A Receipt for a Purging" in 1743. The key ingredient, commonly known today as ipecac but then also known to settlers as "Indian physic," was new to the English upon their arrival in North America. The recipe as Randolph records it, however, fails to acknowledge any Indigenous person as its source, instead crediting a "J. Coupland" for sharing it with her.[51] As Leni Sorensen points out, Randolph's manuscript makes this neglect of non-white sources part of her methods, whether perpetuating the erasures of those who came before her or in introducing new omissions. Even though Randolph enslaved at least thirty-one people at the time of her death in 1766, she also completely obscures their work in her Virginia kitchen.[52] While instances of crediting the work of Black and enslaved people in English and American medical writings certainly exist, these attributions are few and far between in manuscript recipe collections.[53] The Saffin-Ellis manuscript compilation, which likely crossed the Atlantic to a new home in England in the mid-eighteenth century, offers one notable example: a recipe entitled

50 In her discussion of European printings of Nicholas Monardes's influential accounts of New World medical knowledge, Rankin argues that translators "used the archive of practice not to recognize indigenous practitioners but to shore up the authority of European communities against threats both local and foreign." See Alisha Rankin, "New World Drugs and the Archive of Practice: Translating Nicolás Monardes in Early Modern Europe," *Osiris* 37 (2022): 71. As Gabriel puts it, "Indian knowledge of healing plants was thus incorporated into the development of both European and colonial medicine in a way that extracted plants out of Indian cosmologies, reified them as discrete physical things, and transformed them into therapeutic objects that were knowable through the evolving epistemological practices of Western medical science." See Joseph M. Gabriel, "Indian Secrets, Indian Cures, and the Pharmacopoeia of the United States of America," in *Drugs on the Page: Pharmacopoeias and Healing Knowledge in the Early Modern Atlantic World,* eds. Matthew James Crawford and Joseph M. Gabriel, 247.

51 See Randolph's recipe book as reproduced in Katherine E. Harbury, *Colonial Virginia's Cooking Dynasty* (Columbia: University of South Carolina Press, 2004), 418 and Harbury's commentary, xviii. "Indian physic" is mentioned in discussions of gout in chapter 5 of this volume as well; for details on the plant's uses and other names, see Gabriel, "Indian Secrets, Indian Cures, and the Pharmacopoeia of the United States of America," 244.

52 Leni Sorensen, "Keeping a Good House," *Gastronomica* 5, no. 4 (2005): 106.

53 Many scholarly efforts to recover voices of the enslaved in manuscript recipes have concentrated on food preparation. Deetz's study of enslaved cooks acknowledges the overlap with medical expertise, particularly when that knowledge was interpreted as a reason to suspect poisoning. See Kelley Fanto Deetz, *Bound to the Fire: How Virginia's Enslaved Cooks Helped Invent American Cuisine* (Lexington: University Press of Kentucky, 2017), 93–98. Meanwhile, an enslaved physician named Nassaw worked in Virginia with Landon Carter, who recorded in his diary Nassaw's preparation and administration of largely traditional European cures. See Christopher M. Blakley, "'I have been obliged to Send Nassaw': An Enslaved Healer's Medical Labour and Skill in Eighteenth-Century Virginia," *Medical History* 65, no. 2 (2021): 121–39.

"The Negro Caeser's Method of Cure for poison." The compiler, however, quickly signals distance from the Black creator, noting the recipe originated "from the Carolina gazet in America."[54] And indeed, the manuscript keeper could have encountered the recipe in one of its many reprintings in London periodicals in 1750, rather than directly from an American source.[55]

Traveling Recipes: Ingredients in England

When English settlers crossed the Atlantic, they relied upon healthcare recipes derived from English surroundings, offering long-established cures for humorally similar bodies suffering from ailments generated within more familiar environments. These recipes often proved ineffective and difficult to produce in North America, yet the manuscript compilers who lived there often clung to these inherited treatments and their associations of English identity and bodily health. At the same time, necessity drove them to adopt new healthcare practices, principally learned originally, if not directly, from unnamed Indigenous peoples. As Gabriel notes, standard practices came to reflect this process of adoption without attribution, "simply based on the number of plants with the name 'Indian' in their colloquial name that appeared in medical texts printed in both the colonies and the early United States, including Indian physic, Indian pink, Indian poke, Indian lettuce, Indian turnip, Indian paint, Indian cucumber, Indian sage, and Indian tobacco (or lobelia)."[56]

The ingredients and knowledge gleaned from American sources soon crossed the ocean to Europe, where they blended with materials with

54 *Saffin-Ellis Miscellany*, 1716–1762, University of Pennsylvania Ms. Codex 230, 176r. As we shall see in chapter 5, copying newspaper recipes into manuscript recipe books becomes common practice, especially in the early eighteenth century. For more on this practice of recording newspaper recipes in family manuscripts, see Leong, *Recipes for Everyday Knowledge*, 147–72.
55 While the Saffin-Ellis recipe references a South Carolina newspaper, Morgan points out that Ceaser's recipe also appeared in London magazines like *The Gentleman's Magazine* and *The London Magazine*, as well as several North American publications. See Philip D. Morgan, *Slave Counterpoint* (Chapel Hill: University of North Carolina Press, 1998), 628. Morgan does not link the recipe to the Saffin-Ellis collection, but that manuscript's recipe seems connected to this enslaved man, who was freed in recognition of his medical skills. The Saffin-Ellis manuscript refers to the *Gentleman's Magazine* in several recipes (see "An account of the Inward use of Nightshad" in the *Saffin-Ellis Miscellany*, 1716–62, University of Pennsylvania Ms. Codex 230, 167r which references the September 1757 edition of the publication), and indeed "The Negro *Caeser*'s Cure for Poison" appears in a 1750 issue of *Gentleman's Magazine*; see "The Negro *Caeser's* Cure for Poison," *Gentleman's Magazine and Historical Quarterly* 20 (1750): 342–43.
56 Gabriel, "Indian Secrets, Indian Cures," 244.

better-known histories. While they may not have directly considered what imported ingredients might do to their bodies, English recipe compilers were aware of the transformational impacts that cures from America and other outposts brought for healthcare. Ingredients in manuscript compilations could originate from the other side of the globe or from a neighboring field and wind up in the same English medical recipe, where their distinct qualities balanced each other to match the sufferer's bodily needs. As we shall see, botanical ingredients could be shipped from rural communities to urban centers within England, and imported spices from far-off ports moved along country roads to apothecary shops in rural Yorkshire towns. In her survey of recipe compilations, in print and manuscript, Anne Stobart finds that more than 38 percent of ingredients could have been obtained at a local apothecary in England, disconnected from their sources and prepared for sale.[57] Whether imported from abroad or obtained from English fields and gardens, the number of ingredients sold through apothecary shops underscores the connections between domestic medicine and commercial forces—forces that, as we shall see in the case of rheumatism, also influenced the labels that recipe compilers attached to the diseases and symptoms they encountered.

As they listed the ingredients and sources for their entries, compilers of manuscript recipe collections at times sketched out vague maps of their recipes' beginnings, revealing tantalizing glimpses of their homes, as well as their social networks and travel histories in the process. In the case of collections inherited by family members, manuscript origins and travels can seem obvious, especially since, in many such cases, compilers helpfully include the names of those who have shared their recipes. When they attribute recipes to family members, they create sketches of the concerns common among their kin. Similarly, attributions hint at the social connections and access to professional care that a given compiler might enjoy. Yet many attributions prove far murkier, offering names whose connection to the compiler remains elusive. As Michelle DiMeo argues, attributions constitute "vague tag[s]," which could indicate where a recipe originated, though "it could also be that the compiler received [a recipe] from an unnamed intermediary or copied it from a friend's manuscript."[58] Oftentimes, such names cannot be traced at all. But even when no connection can be mapped between a named source and a compiler, the extra effort required to record an attribution points to its perceived significance. In these cases,

57 Stobart, *Household Medicine*, 83.

58 DiMeo, "Authorship and Medical Networks," 27.

the distance from the named origin is often the point, underscoring exactly how far the recipe has traveled to arrive on a given collection's pages. Even when compilers offered no attribution, the recipes they recorded offer a sense of the medical conditions they encountered, or imagined they might encounter, and what combinations of ingredients they considered likely cures in their environments. As compilers learned of new ingredients and came to consider new procedures as possible cures, they included them to have instructions at the ready when the need arose. In that sense we can see the collections covering new territory simply by naming new conditions and by incorporating newly available materials like sassafras and China root. Even if their direct, physical experience of different geographical regions remained unchanged, these books reflect an expansion of the compilers' vision of the interaction with the physical world. They can imagine China root working in their bodies and see a need for cures to new afflictions.

In short, these manuscript collections, and the recipes within them, prove anything but static, embedding within their medicinal cures hints of their movement through space and time. Even when captured on the page, recipes continued to shift and evolve as the books' users made notes and emendations to their texts. Leong furnishes a valuable example of such revision in her study of the Okeover/Adderly family, which "tended to be vocal about tried and tested recipes," making notes for future reference, and for future readers. Such marks transform what might at first seem stable texts into actively evolving sites of experimentation, showing how recipes were "tested, experienced, and customized."[59] And in the case of many manuscript compilations, recipes continued to arrive on their pages, with additions appearing not just on the book's later sections but sandwiched into earlier ones as well.[60] While some recipe manuscripts remain unaltered, with writing all in one hand and clearly delineated sections for cookery and medicine, most contain newly added material, often incorporated without regard to any previous organizational structure. Often in use for generations, many collections include the handwriting of mothers, daughters, and sometimes granddaughters, with later users adding their own recipes and modifying those that earlier writers had recorded.

The raw materials incorporated in healthcare recipes highlight the consequences of a different kind of mobility, as a wider array of medicinal ingredients often became available through growing trade networks. While

59 Leong, *Recipes for Everyday Knowledge*, 91, 101.

60 Jennifer Munroe et al., "Reconstructing Recipes, Recovering Losses, Telling Stories," *Early Modern Studies Journal* 8 (2022), 5–7.

the importation of culinary ingredients widened the pleasures available to English palates, the arrival of new medical cures reminded of the body's susceptibility to the environmental changes brought with travel. As we shall see, recipe compilers in England's north had long mixed local herbs with imported spices in their cures, just as Londoners blended plants from the country with goods they could purchase at apothecary shops. Even when manuscripts stayed put, the recipes written within them increasingly bear the marks of contact with people from around the globe. The importation of goods into London, from European trading hubs, and later from English colonies overseas changed domestic medicine as faraway botanicals became available in country and city alike. English medical knowledge, in the form of recipes and ingredients, flowed to the colonies as well, creating an elaborate give and take between established ways of perceiving not just medical cures but the diseases and conditions they were designed to treat. As new cures arrived to be used on English patients, so did new ideas of what illnesses might exist, and require treatment, in England.

English medicinal recipes thus came to embody a sense of connection to lands and knowledge systems well beyond the local. Indeed, the incorporation of newly available ingredients ran counter to the ideal of self-sufficiency that Gervase Markham espoused in his enormously popular printed household manuals, where he proclaimed that the ideal housewife should rely "more from the prouision of her owne yarde, then the furniture of the markets."[61] Like culinary recipes, knowledge used in preparing medicinal cures traveled from person to person, and in both cases new ingredients often accompanied that transmission of knowledge. Imported medical ingredients rarely proclaim their faraway origins for the benefit of the modern reader, but, for early modern compilers, the arrival of ingredients from the Americas often came with not just an awareness of scarcity but with stories of Europeans suffering from previously unknown illnesses in these far-off lands. Even if newly imported plants like sassafras and guaiacum could treat these afflictions, these new curatives came loaded with significance, and a new sense of physical vulnerability. The

61 Gervase Markham, *Countrey Contentments or The English Husvvife* (London: 1615), 4. This passage has garnered a great deal of attention, notably from Kim F. Hall, "Culinary Spaces, Colonial Spaces: The Gendering of Sugar in the Seventeenth Century," in *Feminist Readings of Early Modern Culture: Emerging Subjects,* eds. Valerie Traub and M. Lindsay Kaplan (Cambridge: University of Cambridge, 1996), 182; Gitanjali G. Shahani, *Tasting Difference: Food, Race, and Cultural Encounters in Early Modern Literature* (Ithaca: Cornell University Press, 2020), 33; and Wendy Wall, *Staging Domesticity: Household Work and English Identity in Early Modern Drama* (Cambridge: Cambridge University Press, 2002), 39–41.

familiar modes of treating ailing English bodies, in short, would no longer suffice.

Considering Recipes in Place

This book contains five chapters, each focusing on recipes in manuscript form that illustrate a distinct, traceable pattern of travel. Each recipe or recipe manuscript illustrates its own blend of knowledge traditions, ingredients, and cultural values, modified as the text moves from place to place. Using feminist and ecocritical approaches, while also calling on recent historical work on early modern commerce and colonial expansion, I explore how the medical knowledge in these recipes and manuscript compilations integrate newly encountered ingredients and practices into long-established healthcare methods. Manuscripts rooted in the English countryside are used to expand what is often a London-centered view of healthcare, revealing how international trade affected domestic medicine in rural areas. As imported ingredients became more available in the countryside, ingredients from faraway locations gradually made their way into previously distinctly rural local practices.

Chapter 1, "Local Waters and Notions of Home in Early Modern Recipe Manuscripts," foregrounds perceived connections between individual bodies and the environments they occupy—concepts that are key to the book's consideration of mobility's impact on early modern healthcare practices. Recipes in manuscript collections often call for specific sorts of water—for example, spring water, "running" water, conduit water, or well water—that would not be available in all locations. This demand for a specific water not only shows awareness that different places provided different raw materials; it also reinforces traditional notions rooted in the Hippocratic treatise *Airs, Waters, Places* that an individual's place of birth influences bodily constitution and therefore determines where a person can experience optimal health. Despite this, manuscripts routinely incorporate a wide variety of specifically named, unprocessed waters, thus suggesting that their owners recognized, and often embraced, the peculiarities of different locations, and acknowledged the adjustments required when moving from place to place. The Downing/Layfield manuscript (College of Physicians of Philadelphia 10a214) provides a vivid example of this urge to record and use cures developed in unfamiliar English places, and to make these cures when separated from the water sources found at home.

The second chapter investigates how medical practices in manuscript recipe collections reflect knowledge gleaned through domestic travel between rural locations and city centers. "'North and South and Middle Countries are Proud in this Lady': Lady Grace Castleton's Recipes and Women's Mobility" examines how Lady Grace Castleton's recipe manuscript reflects her journeys beyond her native Yorkshire. The earliest recipes in *The Lady Grace Castleton's Booke of Receipts* (Folger MS V.a.600) feature the fresh morning milk and bushels of fruit easily accessible in the rural surroundings of her birth, but she also incorporates ingredients from abroad, available to her through travels to London, or even from Yorkshire merchants. The manuscript's recipe for "A Green Ointment" provides a valuable example in its blending of fresh rural ingredients and imported medicinal compounds available most immediately from apothecary shops. I conclude that Lady Castleton's manuscript illustrates how her rural and city homes allowed her to combine the resources of urban and local markets with those of bucolic fields and farms, creating a distinct domestic medical practice built upon a newly expanded array of materials.

While scholars have addressed the impact of diplomatic travels on Ann Fanshawe's recipe collection (Wellcome MS 7113), chapter 3 explores the unacknowledged cosmopolitanism of the recipes Fanshawe inherited from her mother, Margaret Harrison. As the wife of John Harrison, a customs farmer who oversaw activities connected to the London docks, Margaret Harrison had access to a wide variety of imported ingredients, which found their way into Fanshawe's starter recipe manuscript, penned in 1651 by the scribe John Averie. "Considering the Starter Collection: Fanshawe, Family, and Imported Knowledge" argues that Harrison's cures bring an international flavor to Fanshawe's manuscript even before she took it with her to her husband's European diplomatic postings. Comparing recipes Fanshawe attributes to "my mother" with those attributed to her husband's more rurally ensconced relatives, I argue that the Harrison family's London experiences—and the familiarity and availability of new medicinal ingredients that resulted from their trade connections—reveal how the homespun and the international blend in Fanshawe's starter collection, situating it in the world of trade and travel before it ever left England.

Following Margaret Harrison's brother as he sets out across the Atlantic, chapter 4, "Keeping English Bodies: Preserving, Seasoning, and Englishness in Early Virginia Recipes," concentrates on recipes for Dr. Stevens's Water, a home medicine purported to preserve English bodies into a miraculous old age. The recipe arrived early to Jamestown, in the pages of Gervase Markham's *Countrey Contentments*, which the Virginia Company provided to teach inexperienced settler wives established English medical and nutritional practices. Such recipes, however, grated with the realities of disease and hunger in the colony, where food scarcity and unfamiliar climate jeopardized English survival. The physical adjustments settlers underwent threatened to undermine both the ambitions of the new colony and the long-established humoral principles of *Airs, Waters, Places*. The recipe manuscripts that emerged from the new colony's early years—exemplified by those kept by members of the Randolph family—rarely acknowledged these challenges, instead opting to repeat recipes attached to English soil. Such standard, soothing recipes seemed out of sync with widely circulated tales of cannibalism during Jamestown's Starving Time. The enduring appeal of such inherited recipes revealed a yearning to adhere to nationalistic ideas of health and nutrition in a land full of strange plants and diseases.

The book's final chapter, "Traveling Diseases, Imported Cures: Rheumatism and Sassafras in Home Medical Manuscripts," explores the extent to which the need to establish markets for colonial goods influenced ideas of healthcare in English homes. This chapter takes a two-pronged approach in examining the role of sassafras in keeping English colonies in America thriving. America, the chapter shows, was seen as the home of new diseases as well as new cures. Sassafras helped settlers struggle through scurvy and the process of seasoning, but this did little to increase market demand for the plant in England. The Virginia Company's efforts to raise the reputation of sassafras as a medical cure succeeded not just in increasing the plant's appearance in printed medical books; it increased the appearance of certain diseases for it to cure in these manuscripts as well. As recipes requiring sassafras became more common in manuscript collections, that is, so did the appearance of diseases labeled as the "rheumatism" that the plant excelled in curing. Recipe manuscripts like the Frankland family's collection came to incorporate rheumatism as an American disease, one that flourished particularly in the Middle Atlantic and Southeastern colonies. Those who crossed the Atlantic to England brought back not just the disease of rheumatism but its cure, reinforcing but also stretching notions that the places that fostered illnesses provided the most effective cures for those diseases.

Recipe manuscripts illustrate their compilers' habits of accumulating, sorting, and recording knowledge, yet, as the Epilogue shows, they rarely offer the complete picture today's readers might crave. "The Travels of the Great Cordial" explores how early modern practitioners and modern scholars alike have read one of Sir Walter Ralegh's most significant recipes, which survives in his personal papers in manuscript, alongside writings recounting his travels and political troubles. Yet the Great Cordial's extensive ingredient list, incorporating materials from a wide swath of the globe, evolved in the years after Ralegh's death, as domestic compilers and the era's famous scientists worked to establish the recipe's properties. The character of the Great Cordial, in short, remains elusive, despite the powerful public narratives of its travels. Its domestic creation and use retain a sense of the inscrutable, despite the details supplied for its preparation.

Tracing the circulation of knowledge and ingredients in and around England and the American colonies, the chapters that follow examine how recipe manuscripts came to integrate novel ingredients, whether imported from abroad or gathered from nearby lands, and influenced long-established healthcare methods in the process. Individual mobility, and access to recipes and ingredients that traveled, brought new methods and materials to home medical practices, which in turn influenced how families envisioned their relationship to their environment, their bodies, and their nation. Recipes, moreover, traveled in their own right, making homes for themselves in manuscripts maintained by different compilers in vastly different locations. Tracking the movements of a given recipe is often impossible, just as it is impossible as determining the identity of many manuscript compilers. What remains clear is that early modern recipe manuscripts incorporated new ingredients and methods, taking in materials from an expanding world and offering their cures to its furthest known reaches. As they moved, these most domestic of texts reflected, and helped to shape, changing definitions of Englishness.

1. Local Waters and Notions of Home in Early Modern Recipe Manuscripts

Abstract: This chapter uses manuscript recipe references to water to foreground perceived connections between individual bodies and the environments they occupy. Recipes collections often call for specific sorts of water—for example, spring water, "running" water, conduit water, or well water—that would not be available in all locations. This demand for a specific water not only shows awareness that different places provided different raw materials; it also reinforces traditional notions rooted in the Hippocratic treatise *Airs, Waters, Places* that an individual's place of birth influences bodily constitution and therefore determines where a person can experience optimal health. Despite this, the terms used in manuscript recipes often accommodate the adjustments required when moving from place to place.

Keywords: College of Physicians of Philadelphia 10a214; *Airs, Waters, Places*; humors; domestic healthcare; home medicine; water

Water as a natural, rather than symbolic, phenomenon is increasingly making its way into discussions of early modern literature, offering new insights into human interactions with oceans, storms, marshes, rivers, and mineral springs.[1] Investigations of the era's domestic water sources have explored

1 Among the most influential of these works on water writ large are Steve Mentz, *At the Bottom of Shakespeare's Ocean* (London: Continuum, 2009); Lowell Duckert, *For All Waters: Finding Ourselves in Early Modern Wetscapes* (Minneapolis: University of Minnesota Press, 2017); and Hilary Eklund, "Wetlands Reclamation and the Fate of the Local in Seventeenth Century England," in *Ground-Work: English Renaissance Literature and Soil Science*, ed. Hilary Eklund (University Park: Penn State University Press, 2017), 149–70. For a thorough introduction to water control efforts of the era, see Lousie Noble, "A Mythography of Water: Hydraulic Engineering and the Imagination," in *The Palgrave Handbook of Early Modern Literature and Science*, eds. Howard Marchitello and Evelyn Tribble (London: Palgrave, 2017), 445–64. Recent studies of mineral springs as both health and social phenomena appear in Amanda Herbert, *Female Alliances:*

Nunn, Hillary M. *Recipes on the Move in Early Modern England and British North America: Domestic Medicine, Mobility, and Manuscript Culture*. Amsterdam: Amsterdam University Press, 2025.
DOI 10.5117/9789463723398_CH01

issues of urban access and supply,[2] but studies have not yet followed water into England's private kitchens, where it became part of the food, drink, and medicine that in turn nurtured household members. Domestic recipe manuscripts, however, make clear that early modern households required a great deal of water, and at times these texts offer surprising glimpses into the significance placed on that water's source. These manuscripts thus allow us to see how households not only used water, but also how they envisioned it as a key ingredient. The qualities of different waters mattered, and recipes in manuscripts are often careful to note whether water should come from a spring, cistern, or pump. Specifying the type of water to be used is particularly important when producing medicinal treatments, which were commonly described alongside culinary dishes in these domestic manuscripts.[3] This conscientious naming of specific types of unprocessed water in turn underscores the importance not just of the methods but the optimal environments required for the recipes' production. While the recipes themselves may be portable—and indeed these bits of domestic knowledge circulated through wide-ranging social, political, and

Gender, Identity, and Friendship in Early Modern Britain (New Haven: Yale University Press, 2014) and Thomas Willard, "Testing the Waters: Early Modern Studies," in *Bodily and Spiritual Hygiene in Medieval and Early Modern Literature: Explorations of Textual Presentations of Filth and Water*, ed. Albrecht Classen (Berlin: De Gruyter, 2017), 568–94.

2 Valuable studies by Harris, Hardin, Jenner, and Kok concentrate on water in the city, but generally stop at the household door. See Jonathan Gil Harris, "This Is Not a Pipe: Water Supply Incontinent Sources, and the Leaky Body Politic," in *Enclosure Acts*, ed. Richard Burt (Ithaca: Cornell University Press, 1994), 203–28; William Hardin, "'Pipe-Pilgrimages' and 'Fruitfull Rivers': Thomas Middleton's Civic Entertainments and the Water Supply of Early Modern London," *Renaissance Papers* (1993): 63–74; Mark Jenner, "From Conduit Community to Commercial Network? Water in London, 1500–1725," in *Londinopolis: Essays in the Cultural and Social History of Early Modern London c. 1500–c. 1750*, eds. Paul Griffiths and Mark S. R. Jenner (Manchester: Manchester University Press, 2000), 250–72; and Su Mei Kok, "'How Many Arts from Such a Labour Flow': Thomas Middleton and London's New River," *Journal of Medieval and Early Modern Studies* 43, no. 1 (2013), 173–90.

3 Scholarly work on the nature of manuscript recipe compilations has blossomed in recent years. For valuable insights into the medical contents of these manuscripts, see Elaine Leong, *Recipes for Everyday Knowledge* (Chicago: University of Chicago Press, 2018) and Anne Stobart, *Household Medicine in Seventeenth-Century England* (London: Bloomsbury, 2016), as well as Michelle DiMeo and Sara Pennell, eds., *Reading and Writing Recipe Books, 1500–1800* (Manchester: Manchester University Press, 2013); several valuable readings of medicinal recipes appear in Rebecca Laroche and Jennifer Munroe, eds., *Ecofeminist Approaches to Early Modernity* (New York: Palgrave, 2011) as well. For more on the culinary aspects of recipe manuscripts, see Wendy Wall, *Recipes for Thought: Knowledge and Taste in the Early Modern Kitchen* (Philadelphia: University of Pennsylvania Press, 2015), as well as David B. Goldstein and Amy L. Tigner, *Culinary Shakespeare: Staging Food and Drink in Early Modern England* (Pittsburgh: Duquesne University Press, 2016).

kinship networks—the ingredients needed to produce medicinal cures are often available only in specific settings.[4] References to different types of water in domestic recipe manuscripts may help us determine not just where a recipe originates, but what environment a compiler inhabits—perhaps at the moment she copies a list of ingredients into her collection from a friend's manuscript, or at the time when she turns to her book to find an appropriate cure for her patient. As a result, water classifications can reveal the impact that movement from one household to another brought for early modern recipe compilers. Stipulations about what kind of water is needed for recipes also help us to reconstruct the effects that natural and commercial spaces surrounding different homes could exercise over the development of recipe collections. As we shall see, these recipe manuscripts often build in evidence of their owners' ability to adapt to new locations. This sensitivity to physical mobility is indicated in recipe compilations even though they carry traces of the traditional Hippocratic notion that an individual's place of birth influences bodily constitution and therefore determines where a person can experience optimal health. Using College of Physicians of Philadelphia manuscript 10a214 (CPP 10a214) as a case study, this chapter shows how water in recipe manuscripts reveals the important function of both physical location and social networks in early modern domestic practice.

Water has largely been absent from recent studies of early modern recipe ingredients,[5] no doubt because of its assumed omnipresence, but the details these manuscripts supply make clear that not all waters are perceived as equal. Instead, recipes demand specific kinds of water in the creation of particular medicines. These labels are not naming distilled waters; they

4 For more on the significance of attribution and its relationship to recipe assessment, see Sara Pennell, "Perfecting Practice?: Women Manuscript Recipes and Knowledge in Early Modern England," in *Early Modern Women's Manuscript Writing: Selected Papers from the Trinity/Trent Colloquium*, eds. Victoria E. Burke and Jonathan Gibson (Basingstoke: Ashgate, 2004), 250–51 and Michelle DiMeo, "Authorship and Medical Networks," in *Reading and Writing Recipe Books, 1550–1800*, eds. Michelle DiMeo and Sara Pennell (Manchester: Manchester University Press, 2013), 25–46.

5 Most notably, Stobart offers a spectacularly detailed discussion of the ingredients occurring in early modern recipe manuscripts, tracing significant patterns that emerge among recipes with and without donor names, as well as among those with men, rather than women, named as the recipe source. Water is not included in her list of ingredients, however. See Stobart, *Household Medicine in Seventeenth-Century England*, 79–102. Like Stobart, Kowalchuk provides a helpful list of ingredients commonly found in recipe manuscripts, but "water" does not appear among its items. See Kristine Kowalchuk, *Preserving on Paper: Seventeenth-Century Englishwoman's Receipt Books* (Toronto: University of Toronto Press, 2017), 315–58.

instead indicate the sources where water, as a raw material, should be obtained. Recipes often call specifically for "running" or "spring" water, at times further describing this water as "fair"; less often, they require "fountain," "pump," or "conduit" water. These descriptors indicate knowledge of the unique qualities of these different ingredients, implying that water served a vital role in a recipe's effectiveness. The tendency to name specific waters as ingredients when donor names are associated with recipes, moreover, suggests that these cures can be seen as emerging from locations with access to that particular variety of water. Different waters, in short, may signal different characteristics in a recipe's place of origin, or offer clues as to the type of location where the latest modifications to its text were recorded.

The careful recording of descriptors attached to water, moreover, suggests a continued recognition of long-held, classical medical understandings regarding its properties and purity. While English manuscript recipe books may not acknowledge classical traditions where water designation is concerned, these compilations nonetheless incorporate modes of describing water aligned with Hippocratic philosophies, passed down through medical texts still central to medical training in places like Padua and Montpellier. In particular, the principles of the Hippocratic treatise *Airs, Waters, Places*—with its insistence that the qualities of a given physical environment play a formative role in the bodies of those living within it—undergird much of the thinking about the water used in medicinal recipes. Not only did particular qualities permeate the water in different places, the bodies of individuals living in those places were shaped by the vicissitudes of that water. The increasingly mobile nature of early modern England's population, however, required practitioners of domestic medicine to adapt their recipes for use with water sources available in new locales. In naming specific sources for water, domestic manuscript compilations thus reinforced ancient notions of water's particular, local properties, even when they reflect changes in availability in both metropolitan and rural areas.

The Place of Water in Recipe Manuscripts

This study began with experiments involving searchable transcriptions from three manuscripts found in the Folger Shakespeare Library and encoded by members of the Early Modern Recipes Online Collective (EMROC).[6] Word

6 For more on the EMROC collective's transcription work, see https://emroc.hypotheses.org and Laroche et al., "Becoming Visible: Recipes in the Making," *Early Modern Women* 13,

counts in manuscripts owned by Rebeckah Winche, Mary and Timothy Cruso, and one unnamed compiler reveal that *water* ranks among the five most commonly occurring words in each recipe collection.[7] Since these initial explorations, I have factored in word counts from transcriptions of two other manuscripts, the first a collection owned by Mary Granville and passed on to her daughter Ann Granville Dewes, and the second from a College of Physicians of Philadelphia manuscript begun by Calybute Downing before coming into Anne Layfield's possession.[8] Water appears among the top five words in these manuscripts as well. The numbers make water's significance clear in the early modern domestic scene; aside from acting as a key ingredient in medical and cookery recipes, it serves as a tool in preparation and a label for numerous household distillations.[9] Water, in short, permeates such texts, and the attention to its varieties suggests an acknowledgment of its importance in creating effective cures.

Because recipe books were often passed from generation to generation in a single family, and added to by each new owner, these documents show the effects of marriages, social upheavals, technological changes and—particularly important here—their compilers' moves to new residences. These manuscripts shed light on the connections that individual households forged with their surroundings—whether in the form of kitchen gardens, neighboring estates, or even foreign countries—through

no. 1 (2018): 133–43. An increasing number of transcribed recipe manuscripts are available for searching through the Folger Shakespeare Library's online collections, thanks to the combined efforts of EMROC and the Early Modern Manuscripts Online project.

7 *Take* and *put* are the big winners, appearing most frequently in all the manuscripts. See Rebeckah Winche, *Receipt Book of Rebeckah Winche*, c. 1666, Folger MS V.b.366, Folger Shakespeare Library, Washington, DC; Mary Cruso and Timothy Cruso, *Cookbook of Mary Cruso and Timothy Cruso*, 1689, Folger MS X.d.24, Folger Shakespeare Library, Washington, DC; and *Cookbook*, ca. 1720, Folger MS W.b.653, Folger Shakespeare Library, Washington, DC.

8 See the Granville Family, *Cookery and Medical Receipts of the Granville Family, c. 1640–c. 1750*, Folger MS V.a. 430, Folger Shakespeare Library, Washington, DC, also transcribed in Kowalchuk, *Preserving on Paper*, 61–154. The Historical Medical Library at the College of Physicians of Philadelphia catalogs Manuscript 10a214 with *Manuscript Recipes: A Very Interesting MS. Volume of Medical and Household Recipes* in the title field, dating it at c. 1640 (the date that appears next to Anne Layfield's name on the fly-leaf), see Anne Layfield, *Manuscript Recipes: A Very Interesting MS. Volume of Medical and Household Recipes*, c. 1640, CPP 10a214, College of Physicians of Philadelphia, Philadelphia, PA.

9 Recipes for pickles, for example, commonly call for vegetables to be rinsed in several "waters," or, in other words, submerged in several different vats of fresh water. The word *water* also refers to the product of recipes; distilling rose petals, for example, often requires no water, but the resulting rosewater is key to an astonishing number of recipes. Manuscripts like Winche's devote whole sections to distilled waters, which were then in turn used in foods or medical recipes. See Winche, *Receipt Book of Rebeckah Winche*, c. 1666, Folger MS V.b.366.

the foods and medicines they produced and consumed, and often reflect changes in those relationships when individual owners moved to new households. Neatly transcribed "starter collections" of family recipes often accompanied women as they took up new residences upon marrying; in the years, and sometimes generations, that followed, women revised these recipes and added new ones to reflect changes in their surroundings and domestic practices.[10] While men compiled recipes and contributed to household books, these manuscripts have proven particularly useful for the views they provide into the lives of women of various ranks as they performed their domestic duties.[11] As Sara Pennell puts it, evidence of male involvement in recipe compilation does not "render manuscript recipe collections invalid as a means through which to study female knowledge formation. It simply reiterates that, as with other manuscript genres, recipe collections were no more single-source, single-authored, single-generation volumes, than they were destined for a single purpose."[12] The manuscripts thus illuminate the domestic practices of women and their families, highlighting domestic experiences that are often under-represented in scholarly studies.

In the five recipe manuscripts named above, 184 recipes call for water—that is, water that is not a distilled product, such as rosewater or an on-hand, previously prepared medicine like Dr. Stevens's Water.[13] Of these 184 entries that use water as an ingredient, thirty-four, or 18 percent, name the person who shared the recipe with the compiler. What is more striking, however, is that of this subset of thirty-four recipes with attributions—that is, that name a person as the source of a recipe—twenty-four recipes are careful to specify what variety of water should be used, leaving only ten that name water without including a modifier. That means that, in this sample, 71 percent of recipes that carry attributions and demand water are careful to specify where that water comes from, or what qualities it should have. Of

10 See Leong, *Recipes for Everyday Knowledge*, 22–23 and Elaine Leong, "Collecting Knowledge for the Family: Recipes, Gender, and Practical Knowledge in the Early Modern English Household," *Centaurus* 55 (2013): 90–93.

11 See in particular Herbert's examination of recipe collections as illustrations of women's collaborative work in Herbert, *Female Alliances*, 102–16. Examining her handlist of early modern recipe books, Stobart concludes that roughly one third "are attributed to men or unspecified" as to their compiler's identity. See Stobart, *Household Medicine in Seventeenth-Century England*, 30.

12 Pennell, "Perfecting Practice?," 242.

13 Here, I must stress that, though these numbers derive from a limited number of transcribed texts, these trends have remained consistent even as the number of searchable transcriptions has grown. For more on Dr. Stevens's Water, see chapter 4 of this volume.

the 150 recipes without attributions, only fifty-nine, or 39 percent, specify what sort of water is to be used.[14]

The common practice of using previously existing recipe texts as a basis for new household manuscripts contributes to the habit of specifying what water should go into a particular preparation. Keepers of household recipes often copied verbatim from their sources in their drive to acquire new cures from family members, friends, neighbors, medical practitioners, and printed books. In the process, compilers incorporated the specific demands and practices of people who lived elsewhere, and who may have had easier access to different ingredients. While Pennell suggests the creation of recipe manuscripts depended on the "relatively circumscribed familial and geographical nature of [their owners'] networks,"[15] the attention to recording a recipe's demand for a specific water suggests a recognition of different qualities in this essential ingredient. Compilers might record, as Granville does, a cure for a mouth water to treat "any Inflamation or swelling" that calls for conduit water, even if their location has no ready access to a conduit.[16] This might reflect an urge to prepare for unforeseen changes in circumstances—the compiler might anticipate one day living near a conduit, perhaps because of a move or a local improvement—or she might encounter a friend who is in need of such a recipe and would thereby help by passing it on. The compiler, too, might see such a recipe as a good starting point for modification for use within her own circumstances.

Embedded in these recipes, then, is a recognition that different locations and resources affect the medicines that can be produced in individual kitchens. When a compiler records the name of a recipe's donor alongside its instructions, the attribution marks a previous location for the recipe's preparation. This location may not be easily ascertainable for modern readers, as recipe donors can shift residences due to marriage, a change in fortune, or even a change in season, and the names attached to recipes are not themselves always traceable in existing historical records. Nonetheless,

14 On the whole, approximately 45 percent of recipes specify the sorts of water to be used, while 55 percent do not. The number of transcribed texts is growing rapidly, thanks to crowdsourcing work of EMROC, the Folger Shakespeare Library, and volunteers around the globe, and rough searches of these expanded collections suggest that the pattern holds. As Rosvally's recent work has shown, recipes for medicinal cures are even more likely to require a particular source for their unprocessed water. See Danielle Rosvally, "Sifting and Sorting: An Introduction to Database Methods and Pedagogy using Humanist Texts," *Early Modern Studies Journal* 9 (2019).

15 Pennell, "Perfecting Practice?," 245.

16 See Granville Family, *Cookery and Medical Receipts of the Granville Family, c. 1640–c.1750*, Folger MS V.a. 430, 166r, which suggests spring water would be a viable option; transcribed in Kowalchuk, *Preserving on Paper*, 124.

the presence of a donor's name offers clues to the compiler's knowledge network and surroundings. When a doctor's name is invoked, moreover, an attribution can bring onto the domestic scene the medical profession's notions regarding the human body's functions, even if these academic viewpoints are not overtly stated. Thus, when Pennell observes that "appending a donor's name to a recipe served not only to authenticate the distance traveled by a recipe, but also authenticated the particular experience of the donor,"[17] she is highlighting the recipe's traversal of not just physical space but of different realms of medical knowledge and social status before its arrival in a given manuscript.

Water in Flux

As Jonathan Gil Harris argues, London's increasingly sophisticated water system made the city itself seem like the origin of its water supply. Elaborately constructed cisterns and conduits disguised the fact that the water itself usually came from springs beyond the city's boundaries. In that sense, the system of cisterns—and the eventual construction of the New River in 1613, which diverted an entire waterway for Londoners' use—endorsed as well as complicated notions of water as a foundational element of the city's body. London, Harris argues, relied on the illusion of firm boundaries to create the desirable image of a classical, self-contained body politic; the extramural water sources, however, underscored the reality that the civic body not only relied on external resources but also needed to expel unclean water from a system it worked to think of as closed.[18]

Whether in a city or country setting, however, making water available within the household was often considered women's work. The water-hauling efforts of women (whose bodies Gail Kern Paster famously labels as "leaky vessels"[19]) kept the city going, and women surround cisterns and

17 Pennell, "Perfecting Practice?," 251.

18 Indeed, London is the central focus for most scholarly treatments of water supply in the era, and, perhaps unsurprisingly, a fair proportion of that work concentrates on the disposal of sewage. See Harris, "This Is Not a Pipe" as well as Christopher D. Foley, "Marlowe's *Edward II* and 'The Woful Lamentations of Jane Shore': Tactical Engagements with Sewers in Late-Elizabethan England," *Early Modern Literary Studies* 23 (2014) and Julian Yates, *Error, Misuse, Failure* (Minneapolis: University of Minnesota Press, 2003).

19 Paster argues that "cultural association of women and liquids was so deeply inscribed that it required little empirical support" and that "evidence for an iconology of women as leaky vessels must have seemed undeniable." See Gail Kern Paster, "Leaky Vessels: The Incontinent Women of City Comedy," *Renaissance Drama* 18 (1987): 50.

pumps in historical records. When funding the construction of London's Lamb Conduit, for example, William Lamb furnished 120 pails to neighborhood women "wherewith to carrie and serve water," an occupation that he describes as "an honest shift in living, though somewhat toilsome," so that they might avoid "unthriftines and idlenesse."[20] The work could prove dangerous as well. Carole Rawcliffe's study of Tudor city records reveals that female servants and children often drowned in the course of their water-fetching duties, becoming victims of heavy buckets and strong river currents.[21] Literary works feature few references to the actual transport of water from communal source to household, but those that do commonly associate water-hauling with stereotypically feminine incontinence and gossip. In John Taylor's *Stripping, Whipping, and Pumping, or the Five Mad Shavers of Drury Lane*, the communal pump at Reindeer Court becomes the site of a cosmopolitan ducking ritual, where a group of women held another "under the spout, and pump'd Water upon her, and us'd her more shamefully than it is fit to write of."[22]

Such presentations of household water only reinforce anxieties about water's tendency to engulf seemingly independent entities and amalgamate them with one another. Water, after all, ignores boundaries by its nature, seeping into and altering its environs, submerging (and merging together) what it surrounds. It flows—and lies stagnant—in city and country settings alike, containing and carrying materials suspended in it. These qualities are what make water so valuable in both cookery and medicine, allowing distribution of different compounds throughout the body. Ingested and expelled, water complicates ideals of orderliness and the classical body, as Paster and Harris make clear; in a more positive light, it illustrates Nancy Tuana's concept of "viscous porosity," which highlights how "membranes" like "skin and flesh, prejudgments and symbolic imaginaries, habits and embodiments" connect bodily interiors and the surroundings that lie just beyond them.[23] As a result, water epitomizes the idea of the uncontainable, escaping control while binding together the elements it encounters and sweeps along.

20 See Abraham Fleming, *A Memorial of the Famous Monuments and Charitable Almsdeedes of the Right Worshipfull Maister William Lambe* (London, 1580), C3r. Both Harris, "This Is Not a Pipe," 203–28 and Hardin, "'Pipe-Pilgrimages' and 'Fruitfull Rivers,'" 63–74 refer to Lamb's donation.
21 Carole Rawcliffe, *Urban Bodies: Communal Health in Late Medieval and English Towns and Cities* (Woodbridge, Suffolk: Boydell, 2013), 212.
22 John Taylor, *Stripping, Whipping, and Pumping, or the Five Mad Shavers of Drury Lane* (London, 1638), 9.
23 Nancy Tuana, "Viscous Porosity: Witnessing Katrina," in *Material Feminisms*, eds. Stacy Alaimo and Susan Hekman (Bloomington: Indiana University Press, 2008), 200.

With this ability to evade boundaries comes a perceived need for delineation and, as a result, not all early modern waters were considered equal in the era's kitchens. Ideally, waters destined for internal consumption and for use in medications should be drawn from freely running sources, rather than cisterns and pumps, where water stands stagnant. Tobias Venner, a Somerset physician, devotes three pages to the question "Whether fountaine water, in goodnesse and wholsomnesse, excell other waters?"[24] His answer, not surprisingly, is yes, for fountain water is "most cleare and thin, pure in taste and smell"; he ranks rainwater a close second, provided it is gathered in the proper conditions. Water from "pooles, motes, and of pits," should be "eschewed" because "the parching heat of the Sunne" draws off much of its volume and leaves it "corrupted both in smell and taste." The technology of cisterns and pumps does little in Venner's mind to ameliorate the problems associated with stagnation. When all is said and done, "waters that are drawen thorow pumps, because they are shut up from the aire, are worse then other Well-waters, for they more quickly putrifie," and "The like may bee said of Cisternewaters."[25] Yet some preparations explicitly call for water from cisterns or pumps, even though many considered it inferior.

While it is tempting to conclude that designating a certain source for water renders a city recipe distinct from one made in the country, the presence of conduits on rural estates and wells in urban areas quickly dissolves such divisions. At Lady Anne Clifford's Skipton Castle, for example, Conduit Court contained at its center a "great stone basin from which the inhabitants of the castle drew their water, brought into the quadrangle by pipes from a spring three-quarters of a mile away."[26] While such grand systems certainly may not be typical, simple country houses had access to pumps as well—or so Gervase Markham suggests in *The English Husbandman*, where he includes a pump "to serve the offices of the house" in his sketch of the ideal rural home.[27] It is safer to say that examining the varying modifiers applied to water can hint at how compilers used their manuscript recipes in multiple locations, when they found themselves in unfamiliar places and needed to improvise to work with local supplies.

24 The *Oxford English Dictionary* defines "fountain water" as "fresh water from a spring, spring-water" and offers "running water" as a general term in the period for "water taken from a flowing stream or river." See "fountain-water, n.," in *Oxford English Dictionary*, September 23, 2023, and "running water, n." in *Oxford English Dictionary*, July 18, 2023.

25 Tobias Venner, *Via recta ad vitam longam* (London, 1620), 8, 10.

26 George C. Williamson, *Lady Anne Clifford Countess of Dorset, Pembroke & Montgomery* (London: Titus Wilson and Son, 1922), 417.

27 Gervase Markham, *The English Husbandman* (London, 1613), B[1]r.

Water Qualities and Geographical Mobility: A Case Study

The College of Physicians of Philadelphia manuscript 10a214 (CPP 10a214) illustrates the mobility of these handwritten collections while hinting at the varying ingredients available in their different local environments. Though it is difficult to determine where CPP 10a214 was begun or where its multiple compilers lived, we do know that Calybute Downing started the collection before it became the property of Anne Layfield in 1640. The recipes considered here appear in the collection's second half, where one E. Layfield records recipes used by his wife, the Anne Layfield who signed her name in the book. How the collection moved from one owner to the next is not clear, since the Layfield and Downing families share no discernible direct connection by blood or marriage.[28] The mysterious nature of the collection's migration from one household to the next, however, only underscores the tendency of recipes to spring up, without explanation, in unexpected places.

Among the entries in the Layfield pages of the CPP manuscript are two strikingly distinct recipes for curing sores, recorded in the same hand and assuming drastically different access to ingredients—and those modes of access initially make the first recipe seem at home in the country and the second in the city. The recipes appear on pages marked 79 and 82 by an early compiler; they are separated only by one piece of text, a seven-line recipe "To make Excellent Mustard," but they seem to come from different worlds. The first, identified as "a water that will cure any old sore, given to my deare wife by the Lady Ashborneham" is botanically based and requires easy access to rural products as well as to markets where processed ingredients would be available. The second recipe contains a greater proportion of processed or potentially purchased ingredients and suggests less reliance on the natural surroundings as well as greater capacity for accommodating different sorts of locally available water.[29] In short, the two neighboring recipes seem to assume they will be prepared in markedly different surroundings.

28 Rebecca Laroche and I began working to learn more about the Downing and Layfield families in 2012, in Hillary Nunn and Rebecca Laroche, "Exploring Manuscript 10a214," *The Recipes Project*, September 19, 2019, a blog series for *The Recipes Project*. The working hypothesis is that the volume became Layfield property in the 1640s, taking up residence in Essex where Layfield served as a churchman.

29 Layfield, *Manuscript Recipes*, 1640, CPP MS 10a214, College Physicians of Philadelphia, Philadelphia, PA, 79, 82. Stobart's research suggests that medicinal recipes usually required at least one purchased ingredient, although recipes attributed to women were slightly less likely to call for such components. See Stobart, *Household Medicine in Seventeenth-Century England*, 45.

The initial step of the first, more heavily botanical recipe attributed to Lady Ashburnham involves making an herb water, requiring a two-gallon pipkin filled with "Herbe Mercury," gatherred "in the morninge early, & cleane picked, before | it be seeded." Since access to a field in the early morning is much simpler if one lives near it, the recipe suggests a rural setting. Anne Stobart notes that sourcing "wild" ingredients could involve intermediaries even in the country,[30] yet the recipe's phrasing invites readers to imagine Lady Ashburnham, or at least a member of her household, gathering the mercury for immediate use, not just during a prescribed point in the plant's life cycle but at a specific time of day. This insistence on freshness is juxtaposed with the early modern household's routine preservation of seasonal herbs, for the recipe's closing adds, "It is good to make | great store of the herbe-water [produced in the recipe's first steps] without the metals in the | moneth of Aprill or May, for it cannot be made all the | year after."[31] From its opening lines, then, this cure for an old sore is anchored in a household that produces its own herbal waters. A location near a field, or proximity to an herb woman who can deliver these botanical products just after picking them, is essential to proper production.

The water in which the herb mercury is boiled, however, further restricts this first recipe's place of production. It calls for "6 quarts of run- | ninge water, which coms from a Springe that | springeth against the Easte." While this is a manageable quantity of water, not every household would have easy access to such a spring.[32] Given the specific nature of the water's qualities, it is striking that the recipe speaks of the source itself in generic terms, describing its orientation rather than offering a specific spring's name or

30 Layfield, *Manuscript Recipes*, 1640, CPP MS 10a214, 79. Clifford family records, Stobart reveals, show payments for some herbs that could have been easily gathered in local fields, and some plants seem to have been gathered to be sold immediately. See Stobart, *Household Medicine in Seventeenth-Century England*, 87–89.

31 Layfield, *Manuscript Recipes*, 1640, CPP MS 10a214, 79–80. This need for mercury plants that have not gone to seed in April or May suggests that the herb required is English mercury, or Good Henry, which Gerard says flowers in June and July and whose leaves he says are good for "greene wounds, or foule and old ulcers." See John Gerard, *The Herball or Generall History of Plantes* (London, 1633), 329.

32 Layfield, *Manuscript Recipes*, 1640, CPP MS 10a214, 79. How long water taken from a stream can be described as "running" remains unclear—if it is hauled the night before, does it still merit that description? Gordon's comment that "Running water was known at this time to be cleaner and healthier than stagnant or stored water" suggests that the designation cannot apply to water kept in bottles. See Sarah Gordon, "Mens Sana in Corpore Sanus: Water, Wellness, and Cleanliness in Five Fifteenth-Century Medical Manuals," in *Bodily and Spiritual Hygiene in Medieval and Early Modern Literature: Explorations of Textual Presentations of Filth and Water*, ed. Albrecht Classen (Berlin: De Gruter, 2017), 427.

geographical location. Thus, even when some recipe collections pointed users to particular apothecary shops in cities for ingredients, this manuscript offers no particulars about locating this recipe's spring water.[33] Suitable water, it makes clear, can come from *a* spring that faces east, rather than one particular spring. The recipe, in short, builds in its own portability even as it invites readers to imagine Lady Ashburnham in her own distinct rural field—in this case, perhaps her family estate, Ashburnham Place, in Sussex—as she gathers ingredients for the cure.[34]

While CPP 10a214 suggests the possibility of multiple settings for this particular recipe's production, it is nonetheless jarring to see it surface, in nearly identical language, in Johanna St. John's recipe book, where it is labeled "Dr. Sheafs water for an Old sore."[35] Despite the different attribution, the recipe is a near duplicate of the cure E. Layfield records in CPP 10a214, requiring "an earthen Pipkin holding two gallons with the herbe mer | cury gathered e[a]rly in the morning & also before it be seeded," along with "6 quarts of running water out of a spring against the | east." The recipe's appearance in two manuscripts, with different attributions but nearly identical instructions and ingredients, demonstrates the fluidity of recipe circulation, with origins becoming murky even as the knowledge transmitted remains intact. Even though it is attributed to Dr. Sheaf rather than Lady Ashburnham, the recipe in St. John's book also suggests making "good store of the Herb water in April & may without | the mettles" and offers similarly

33 Herbert, *Female Alliances*, 109–10. Herbert stresses that the exchange of information regarding ingredient sources fostered a sense of security within women who found themselves in unfamiliar urban settings. Advice on imported ingredients proved common as well, and the absence of information on rural ingredients suggests an assumed familiarity with the countryside.

34 The manuscript offers no direct clues as to which Lady Ashburnham provided this recipe, but likely contenders are Elizabeth Beaumont Ashburnham Richardson, *suo jure* baroness of Cramond (1576/7–1651), who is author of the prayer collection *A Ladies Legacie to her Daughters* (1645), or her daughter-in-law Frances Holland Ashburnham (1613–49), wife to her son John. See Burke's entry on Ashburnham in the *Oxford Dictionary of National Biography*, Victoria E. Burke, "Richardson [*née* Beaumont; *other married name* Ashburnham], Elizabeth *suo jure* baroness of Cramond (1576/7–1651)," in *The Oxford Dictionary of National Biography*, Oxford University Press, January 3, 2008, accessed October 31, 2024; along with the Perdita Project's biography, "Perdita Woman: Lady Elizabeth Ashburnham (later Richardson)," *Perdita Project*, accessed September 9, 2019; Heller also offers valuable background on Ashburnham's writing, Jennifer Heller, *The Mother's Legacy in Early Modern England* (Basingstoke: Ashgate, 2011), 71.

35 Johanna St. John, *Johanna St. John her Book*, 1680, Wellcome MS Western 4338, Wellcome Collection, London, England, 210r. A complete transcription of this manuscript is underway through EMROC, but, since it is not yet complete, St. John's manuscript was not included in my word count studies.

detailed instructions for the end product's use.[36] The appearance of this cure for an old sore in two manuscripts underscores the multiple settings in which the recipe can be successfully prepared. We cannot simply picture Lady Ashburnham, or her servants, strolling through the estate's fields on a spring morning to collect the necessary herbs. Indeed, the recipe's appearance in St. John's book conjures a dramatically different image of the recipe's production and origin, adding a London doctor into the mix. Her note suggests that the recipe itself comes not from a rural estate but from an urban source. The most prominent "Dr. Sheaf" of the era, after all, is Thomas Sheaf, who lived in London and played an influential role in the Royal College of Physicians.[37]

The St. John manuscript's recipe for an old sore, then, suggests urban knowledge can seep into the countryside, where makers blend fresh rural plants with processed ingredients from beyond the estate; at the same time, it makes clear that rural expertise streams into the city as well. The recipe's demand for ingredients from the country reflects a typical pattern of transporting fresh ingredients, or perhaps semi-processed cures developed from them, from the rural homestead to the urban setting. The cure, even if prepared and taken in the city, brings its country roots with it, infusing the patient's body with rural botanical goodness in a concentrated liquid form. As Elaine Leong points out, St. John left a trail of letters tracing her movements between her city home in London and Lydiard House, her country estate, detailing the flow of medicinal resources between these rural and urban homes. Living in the city when her husband was engaged in business, St. John routinely wrote her estate's steward, Thomas Hardyman, asking that fresh ingredients like butter and roses be sent to London for her use in making balsams and rosewater, respectively.[38] On the other hand, one letter's instructions on making citron water, accompanied by a supply of the fruits, show that St. John had Lydiard House servants prepare some medicines in the country using ingredients obtained in the city, rather than complete the task

36 St. John tells the user to "apply noe salve" to the sore and instead wash it "with Ducks feathers dipt in the water | & lay on the smooth side of a mercury leafe or a rag | dipt in it"; the CPP manuscript instructs caregivers to "apply no salue to it, onely wash it with a bundell of Ducks-feathers & lay upon the soar the smooth side of a Mercury leafe or alitle [cloth] wetted in the water." See St. John, *Johanna St. John her Book,* 1680, Wellcome MS Western 4338, 210r and Layfield, *Manuscript Recipes*, 1640, CPP MS 10a214.

37 Dr. Thomas Sheaf practiced in London 1628–57. See Margaret Pelling and Frances White, "SHEAF, Thomas," in *Physicians and Irregular Medical Practitioners in London 1550–1640 Database*, London, Centre for Metropolitan History, 2004.

38 Leong, *Recipes for Everyday Knowledge*, 36, 64.

herself in London. The result is a mixture of the rural labor and urban-sourced ingredients, made even more impossible to attach to one particular location when considering the citron water's reliance on imported canary wine.[39]

Even given the demand for freshly picked herb mercury, it would be a mistake to see the CPP and St. John manuscripts' cure for an old sore as reflecting an ideal image of an isolated rural estate. On the contrary, the CPP recipe goes on to call for metals, in the form of "white | sublimed mercury," and "3 quarters of | an ounce of Allame."[40] These materials, it is clear, would require access to a market; in fact, most mercury was imported, and the center of English alum trade was in Yorkshire, quite a distance from the Layfield's Essex home and St. John's estate in Wiltshire.[41] Travel, in other words, is incorporated into this seemingly rural domestic cure, and obtaining its ingredients requires a system of English, and international, trade. And, of course, the testimonials of the recipe's effectiveness rely on its wide travels as well. Before the recipe reached Mrs. Layfield, the CPP manuscript notes, it was tested by "her ladyship's sister" (whether this is Lady Ashburnham's sister or some other lady's kin is not clear).[42] Word of its effectiveness presumably spread from there, through networks that, if nothing else, encompassed ground between the Layfields in Essex and the Ashburnham's family estate in Sussex. How Lady Ashburnham acquired the recipe is unclear as well—did she receive it from Dr. Sheaf or from St. John, or from someone else entirely? Or did she donate the recipe to one of them? The lack of precise dating for these manuscripts—yet alone of the recipes within them—frustrates any attempt to trace the recipe's flow among these various named households, if indeed any direct connections exist. Of course, these individuals may not have known each other at all, and innumerable other unnamed parties could have played a role in the recipe's transmission. The specific water may simply be a remnant of the text from which Lady Ashburnham copied it; as we have seen, recipes with attributions are far more likely to provide details about water sources than those without, so determining the point at which the east-facing

39 Leong, *Recipes for Everyday Knowledge*, 62.

40 Layfield, *Manuscript Recipes*, 1640, CPP MS 10a214, 79.

41 Alum, commonly associated with the dye and leather trades, was used as a styptic to stop bleeding. See Nancy Cox and Karin Dannehl, eds., *Dictionary of Traded Goods and Commodities 1550–1820* (Wolverhampton: University of Wolverhampton, 2007), *British History Online*, accessed September 17, 2019; Stobart and Kowalchuk also include alum in their exceedingly helpful glossaries of early modern medical ingredients. See Kowalchuk, *Preserving on Paper* and Stobart, *Household Medicine in Seventeenth-Century England*.

42 Layfield, *Manuscript Recipes*, 1640, CPP MS 10a214, 79.

spring became essential to the recipe as copied in CPP 10a214 would require examining Lady Ashburnham's recipe manuscript, if only such a text could be found, and her sources as well.[43]

Given the specificity of this first recipe for an old sore, it is striking that the CPP manuscript's second recipe for a similar ailment—"The rare water to cure all soares made by my Deare wife"—presents a notable disregard for its water sources. Even though it appears almost immediately after Lady Ashburnham's water, this second recipe reflects Layfield's awareness of the cure's life within his own household rather than a concern with the specifics of water. The recipe resembles a treatment for "Mormols festures Cankers Ulcers or any other sores," appearing in the CPP manuscript's early pages in a different hand,[44] but makes no acknowledgment of this earlier cure. Instead, the "rare water" made by the writer's "Deare wife" builds in flexibility in its preparation, creating a marked contrast from recipes naming donors from beyond the household. The recipe calls for a powder of rock alum and green copperas, two ingredients that necessitate trade and that might make the recipe appear less homespun than the preceding cure for an old sore. In fact, the cure requires no fresh herbs whatsoever; instead, it calls only for ingredients that could be easily found in markets and apothecary shops, or in rural pantries whether in spring or the dead of winter:

> Take Roach Allam one pownd, Greene Copperice halfe
> apound, beate them very small, put them together
> into an Earthen wett glazed pan with a [broad] bottome
> Set them upon the fire, boile them, continually stir-
> ringe them till they be so thicke that you can no
> longer stirr them. Then let them stand till they be
> cold. take them out & beate them to very small powder
> then take pure springe water, or runninge or,
> pumpe water, set it in a posnett (as great or small
> as thow will) upon the fire, till it begin to boyle (&

43 Through personal correspondence, the Senior Archivist of the East Sussex Record Office stated that there are no recipe books associated with the Ashburnham family and their Sussex estate collections, 1048–1984. See Philip Bye, "Ashburnham Recipe Book," email message sent to author, June 20, 2018.

44 The earlier "water for Mormols festures Cankers Ulcers or any other sores" appears on page 8 of the manuscript. It too calls for a pound of rock alum and half a pound of green copperas, and it creates a similar powder. It calls for "fair" water; it does not, however, suggest using plantain water in the later phases, nor does it offer the same cautions about reserving special equipment for the recipe's preparation. See Layfield, *Manuscript Recipes*, 1640, CPP MS 10a214, 8, 79, 82.

> no longer) then take it off the fire, & powr so much
> of the powder presently into the water so longe as it
> makes the water rise or buble up with a hissinge noyse.[45]

The wide array of options for water sources seems jarring after the earlier recipe's insistence on water from an east-facing spring. In fact, the recipe initially can seem rather loose in its requirements, with its options for "pure springe water, or runninge or, | pumpe water," though its precise instructions for handling the metals correct that impression in the lines that follow. While the choice of water seems not to affect to the cure's success, the recipe's phrasing acknowledges that a person preparing it might expect specifics. The maker, in short, was at least familiar with the different sorts of water that could be used; perhaps she even has direct access to this array of sources and might want to remind herself that any would fit the bill. The list of options suggests plentitude, but it may also show an awareness that this plentitude does not always exist and that many available waters would suffice.

This "rare water" for an old sore, in short, seems at first much less attached to a geographical setting than the preceding recipe—it requires no fresh herbs and can be produced in a variety of environments, city or country, in locations supplying only the usually inferior pump water or water drawn from the local stream. The husband recording the recipe, moreover, seems to have had the opportunity to see the recipe produced regularly; he writes, after all, that it was "made by my Deare wife," and he may have known about her adjustments when working in different circumstances. His comment that the medicine "is very hard to [be] done | well, unless it be shewed by one that hath seene it | done" suggests that he has firsthand or even eyewitness knowledge of its production. That impression is furthered by his willingness to offer the following notes to the reader:

> Note 1 that thow fill the posnett halfe with
> pure water, & the other halfe with Plantin water
> if it can be gott 2 that this water so made will
> keepe good a weeke or 14 dayes for your use 3
> when thow use any of it, power alitle of it (as
> much as thow have occasion to use) into a sawcer
> before & warme it on the embers, before thow
> wash the soare with it. 4 dipp alitle cloath in the
> water to wash the soare with. 5 use the same

45 Layfield, *Manuscript Recipes*, 1640, CPP MS 10a214, 82.

sawcer for no other use
whichsoever.[46]

The notes underscore a built-in flexibility in the recipe as well as the skill required in making and administering the cure. The ingredient noted as most difficult to procure, moreover, is plantain water, even though that distilled liquid is a common ingredient in recipes of the period, made from a plant that John Gerard claims "grows almost every where," and even though six other recipes involving plantain occupy the same manuscript.[47] Perhaps his household did not have a reliable source for plantain itself, or the water prepared from it was not regularly available for purchase. Either way, this common ingredient is one that his household, whether in a rural or urban environment, did not always have available for use.

This recipe, however, is far from rootless, despite its seeming disregard for specifics of water that could hint at a particular type of location. The preparation unfolds, after all, in the writer's household, and his own wife is tending the production. The recipe thus establishes his wife, not the setting, as the stable factor in the cure's creation, and her knowledge and practice prove vital in a way that water sources do not. Her skill takes precedent, suggesting a potential for improvisation in her preparation and a resourcefulness that compensates for variability in supplies. In suggesting that the practitioner is the constant—rather than the location and the water found there—this second recipe points to a different mode of describing optimal ingredients for a family's bodily comfort and health. It creates a different sense of home, one where the presence of individuals is identified as more significant than the water available in the surroundings. The effective cure, Layfield suggests, is one made by his wife, rather than one that incorporates waters from one particular place linked to his family's lineage.

Fluid Definitions: Home in the *Airs, Waters, Places* Tradition

The different attitudes toward water in the CPP manuscript's two recipes for curing an old sore highlight varying modes of defining home in early

46 Layfield, *Manuscript Recipes*, 1640, CPP MS 10a214, 82.

47 Gerard uses these words to describe the ubiquity of both land plantain and water plantain. Plantain or plantain water also appear in CPP 10a214's cures for strained sinews, cankers, ulcers in the bladder, chest congestion, and toothaches. See Gerard, *The Herball or Generall History of Plantes*, 421, 418; and Layfield, *Manuscript Recipes*, 1640, CPP MS 10a214, 5, 28, 33, 37, 42, 208.

modern recipe manuscripts, underscoring contrasting perceptions of the relationships between bodies and their physical surroundings. The first recipe's insistence on water from an east-facing spring may at first read as specifically local knowledge, but its requirements also align with traditional medical notions dating back to the ancient world. The Hippocratic treatise on *Airs, Waters, Places* undergirds English understanding of the relationship between individual bodies and their natural environments, positing birthplace as determining where bodies will thrive and where they might suffer. The treatise takes as its starting point the assertion that the composition of human bodies reflects the particular environments they inhabit—an assertion that many have seen as supporting notions of otherness that nurture colonialist thinking.[48] It therefore follows that understanding the qualities of a locale's water is vital to treating its population. According to Jacques Jouanna, the Hippocratic treatise declares that "the properties of spring waters depend principally on the nature of the terrain from which they spring and, secondarily, on their orientation, which can have a positive or negative effect on the qualities necessarily resulting from the terrain. Springs facing east are best; second are springs that face north; third, springs that face west; the most harmful are those that face south."[49] Several sixteenth-century English writers echo this thinking, with Thomas Elyot's *Castel of Health* praising water "whiche issueth out of a spring in the east, and passeth swiftly among great stones or rockes"[50] and Stephen Batman's *Batman uppon Bartholome* declaring, "Savourye water is cléere of substance, of a well that springeth Eastwarde."[51] Venner's later evaluation of the east-facing spring thus calls on a long tradition of English writers, who themselves echo Hippocrates, even if they do not name the

48 For a summary of scholarship linking *Airs, Waters, Places* to colonialist thinking, see Roberto Lo Presti, "Shaping the Difference: The Medical Inquiry into the Nature of Places and the Early Birth of Anthropology in the Hippocratic Treatise *Airs Waters Places*," in *Medicine and Space: Body, Surroundings and Borders in Antiquity and the Middle Ages*, eds. Patricia A. Baker, Han Nijdam, and Karine van't Land (Leiden: Brill, 2012), 174. While Floyd-Wilson does not mention *Airs, Waters, Places* in developing her notion of "geo-humoralism," her discussion of the impact of Galenic non-naturals as influences on ethnological discourse provides a useful parallel. See Mary Floyd-Wilson, "English Mettle," in *Reading the Early Modern Passions: Essays in the Cultural History of Emotion*, eds. Gail Kern Paster, Katherine Rowe, and Mary Floyd-Wilson (Philadelphia: University of Pennsylvania Press, 2004), 113.

49 Jacques Jouanna, "Water, Health and Disease in the Hippocratic Treatise Airs, Waters, Places," in *Greek Medicine from Hippocrates to Galen: Selected Papers*, ed. Philip van der Eijk (Leiden: Brill, 2012), 164.

50 Thomas Elyot, *Castel of Health* (London, 1539), 30.

51 Stephen Batman, *Batman uppon Bartholome* (London, 1582), 80.

Greek sources directly.[52] While Venner applies these ancient principles to his surroundings in Somerset, Lady Ashburnham evokes the standard in Sussex and St. John's Dr. Sheaf brings it to cosmopolitan London circles.

CPP 10a214's and the St. John manuscript's shared cure for an old sore thus grounds itself in classical sources, even though the *Airs, Waters, Places* tradition is not openly acknowledged in any way. Yet many English practitioners explicitly invoked Hippocratic authority to discuss the importance of keeping environment in mind. William Bullein, for example, declared that "A wise phisicion ought to know the natures of men, of waters, of aire, of regions, and dwellings" associated with a "natural English man of birth and education"; he explains that this identity nonetheless incorporates great variety because "our dwellinges in this land, be variable as fennes, marishes, woods, heithes valleis, playnes, and rockie places, and neare the sea side."[53] He holds that England's many landscapes and climates, like those of the ancient world, exercise particular effects on the individuals living in them. "For Hippocrates saieth in his booke of Aire and Water," Bullein reasons, "cities and townes, which are placed toward the east, be more sure, then the townes builded towardes the north, for temperat aire or winde, and sicknesses be lesse. And in the said book *Avicen* greatly commendeth pleasant rivers, running towards the rising of the sunne."[54] Bullein directly connects his assertion to the ancient world, citing both Hippocrates and Avicenna to draw conclusions about water sources mirrored in the CPP/St. John recipe, recognizing no incongruity in applying evaluations of far-off landscapes to English surroundings.[55] Invoking the authority of canonical medical knowledge, he hints at an underlying assumption of similarity among readers and their homes, even as the texts themselves travel from

52 Moffett also endorses the value of east-facing springs, explaining that houses face the east because "all waters and springs running that way, are most clear fragrant pleasant and wholesome." See Thomas Moffett, *Health's Improvement* (London, 1655), 17.

53 William Bullein, *The Government of Health* (London, 1595), 30–31.

54 Bullein, *The Government of Health*, 31. Hart, a Northampton physician, calls upon Hippocrates and Avicenna in an identical fashion, even though his practice is based far away from Bullein's. His detailed discussion of water sources cites the Hippocratic treatise directly, using its Latin name, *de aere, aquis & locis*, and quotes Avicenna's preference for springs "that runne towards the Sunne rising, and have their aspect that way." See James Hart, *Klinike, or The Diet of the Diseased* (London, 1633), 26.

55 Curiously, Bullein makes no mention of the environmental differences that might occur among the many different English locations—ranging from Northumberland to London—where he practiced. See Wallis's entry for Bullein in the *Oxford Dictionary of National Biography*, Patrick Wallis, "William Bullein," in *Oxford Dictionary of National Biography*, Oxford University Press, September 23, 2004, accessed September 9, 2019.

place to place claiming usefulness in the understanding of the human body's inner workings.

How much, given this link between home turf and bodily constitution, could people move without jeopardizing their health? After all, as Andrew Wear puts it, the *Airs, Waters, Places* tradition holds that "the body was made up of the same qualities as climate," so an essential link existed "between people, places, and health."[56] Yet, as Joyce E. Chaplin notes in her discussion of maritime medicine, "If early modern Europeans had really believed themselves to be adapted to specific parts of the world, and at risk of ill health if not death if they left their native 'airs, waters, and place,' then there would be no Western imperial history."[57] Wear points out that the flexibility of these Hippocratic principles allowed colonists a handy way of convincing others to join them abroad. He notes that Thomas Welde, an early Massachusetts Bay colonist, insisted that their North American location "agreeth with our English bodies [so well] that they were never so healthy in their native country."[58] But the physician James Hart, practicing in Northampton, makes an explicit caution about such drastic relocation, calling explicitly on the Hippocratic *Airs, Waters, Places* tradition to do so:

> But because most men must be contented with that aire they first breathed in; therefore this would chiefly be diligently & carefully considered of our new colonies, who transplant themselves into remote regions, that they first make choice of a country, whose naturall temper differeth not much from their owne.[59]

Seafaring and colonial homesteading involve a far more drastic departure from home than moving from England to Italy for medical training, or even moving periodically from the English countryside to London, as many early modern women recipe compilers did. On a smaller scale, though, this potential to adapt household medical practices to non-natal locations offered

56 Andrew Wear, "Place, Health, and Disease: The *Airs, Waters, Places* Tradition in Early Modern England and North America," *Journal of Medieval and Early Modern Studies* 38, no. 3 (2008): 461.

57 Joyce E. Chaplin "Earthsickness: Circumnavigation and the Terrestrial Human Body, 1520–1800," *Bulletin of the History of Medicine* 86 (2012), 516.

58 Wear quotes "Thomas Welde to His Former Parishioners at Tarling, June/July 1632," in *Letters from New England: The Massachusetts Bay Colony 1629–1638*, ed. Everett Emerson (Amherst: University of Massachusetts Press, 1976), 96. See Andrew Wear, "The Prospective Colonist and Strange Environments: Advice on Health and Prosperity," in *Cultivating the Colonies: Colonial States and Their Environmental Legacies*, ed. Christina Folke Ax et al. (Athens, OH: Ohio University Press, 2011), 22.

59 Hart, *Klinike*, 15.

domestic practitioners a wider geographical range to explore when searching for helpful cures, even as it heightened their awareness of the effects that physical location might exercise over the bodies under treatment. Tales of humans successfully adjusting to alien climates, after all, recognize not only the instability that relocation could bring to an individual's health, but also underscore that these changes in health can be countered with proper medical care. Household recipe manuscripts not only illustrate this potential for human mobility; they embody it through their adjustments to the domestic medical practices they record.

Adaptability, Portability, and Recipe Manuscripts

As tenuous as this adaptability of human bodies may be, the largely unspoken assumption that individuals could live in multiple locations explains in part the portability of both recipes and recipes manuscripts. The assumption that individuals could successfully, if not easily, travel between urban and rural homes, not to mention across oceans, offers insight into many manuscript compilers' habitual recording of multiple recipes for a single ailment. While such variations may not proclaim an association with a different geographical location, they make clear that domestic medicine had to make do with what was on hand, and that different ingredients would be available in different places, whether because of trade, seasonal availability, or geographical situation. In that sense, recipe manuscripts reveal a deep awareness that place matters, hinting at their compilers' knowledge through experience and community networks, if not through direct study, of the "airs, waters, and places" tradition.

The CPP manuscript's two recipes for treating an old sore declare drastically different origins and reflect different geographical influences, yet they exist, virtually side-by-side, in the same manuscript. The juxtaposition of these two approaches to water vividly demonstrates that recipes from a wide array of origins often mingle within any given domestic manuscript's pages. While considering manuscripts like CPP 10a214 as independent and coherent collections certainly has merit, the detailed naming of waters on their pages makes clear that the recipes, like London's water, originate from places well beyond the books' pages. The recipes often hail from different geographical locations, though those places are often not easy to pinpoint on a map. Some recipes carefully identify the people and places to which they owe their creation, while others offer incomplete origin stories, if any. At the same time, domestic manuscripts themselves make clear that treating the health condition in question requires active engagement with the local environment and the specific patient's constitution. Some recipes, while not labeled explicitly so, work better for certain bodies, and some recipes can only be produced in certain places. Recipe manuscripts, in other words, build in choices to suit the changing conditions under which their owners work. Those conditions often result from the owners' movements from place to place in the course of their lives, as well as their encounters with the bodies of those who have undertaken travels of their own.

The contents of recipe manuscripts, as a result, prove remarkably fluid, holding in a kind of liquid suspension the interactions—with environments, neighbors, medical authorities, and markets—that give rise to their filled pages. Each recipe in a manuscript suggests a history of local adjustments, and those individual recipes come together to form collections that hint at their wide-ranging origins even as they work to consolidate household knowledge. Full of recipes that float next to one another, these manuscripts allow us to glimpse their connections to lives and places beyond their covers, and beyond the walls of the households where their owners lived. Focusing on water in these manuscripts thus underscores not only that these recipes flowed from person to person, and from place to place; it also challenges us to understand how those eddying forces allow recipes to coalesce in the distinct but often overlapping manuscripts whose significance we are just learning to appreciate today.

2. "North and South and Middle Countries are Proud in this Lady": Lady Grace Castleton's Recipes and Women's Mobility

Abstract: This chapter investigates how medical practices in manuscript recipe collections reflect knowledge gleaned through domestic travel between rural locations and city centers. The earliest recipes in *The Lady Grace Castleton's Booke of Receipts* feature the fresh morning milk and bushels of fruit easily accessible in the rural surroundings of her birth, but her recipes also incorporate ingredients from abroad, available to her through travels to London, or even from Yorkshire merchants. The manuscript's recipe for "A Green Ointment" provides a valuable example of its blending of fresh rural ingredients and imported medicinal compounds available most immediately from apothecary shops, illustrating how Castleton's rural and city homes created her distinct domestic medical practice built upon a newly expanded array of materials.

Keywords: Folger MS V.a.600; Belasyse Family; travel; green ointment; ingredients; recipe circulation

It might seem strange that, as someone supposedly embodying the ideals of domestic stability, Lady Grace Castleton is repeatedly praised upon her death for moving house. The one-page tribute printed as a memorial to her upon her death in 1667, entitled *A Funeral Elegy on the Right Honourable the Lady Viscountesse Castleton*, notes that "Her neighbors found she did the hungry feed" before quickly uprooting her from her surroundings with the following lines: "With her dear Lord she up to London went, / Whence she was call'd to Heav'ns Parliament."[1] While how long and how

1 Jo. Sh., *A Funeral Elegy on the Right Honourable the Lady Viscountesse Castleton* (London, 1667), 1.

Nunn, Hillary M. *Recipes on the Move in Early Modern England and British North America: Domestic Medicine, Mobility, and Manuscript Culture*. Amsterdam: Amsterdam University Press, 2025.
DOI 10.5117/9789463723398_CH02

regularly Lady Castleton lived in London remains unclear, the tribute maps her death as a parallel to her husband George Saunderson's dutiful service in the House of Lords, suggesting she accompanied him to the city four years after their marriage in Yorkshire.[2] The tribute thus attempts a brief positive spin on the movement that is otherwise portrayed as fundamentally wrenching:

> In Yorkshire she was born, in London dead,
> In Lincolnshire her dust lyes buried:
> Thus North and South, and middle Countries are
> Proud in this Lady, each to have a share.[3]

All three locations can claim a piece of Lady Castleton, even if only one of them can serve as her final resting place. Attaching Lady Castleton's identity to these locations, the poet echoes early modern ideas that the constitution of individual bodies reflected the lands they inhabited. In Lady Castleton's case, bodily health decreases with every relocation, as she shifts from "born" in Yorkshire to "dead" in London, to mere "dust" in Lincolnshire. Moving, even in words, damages her bodily integrity, resulting in an odd if poetic tug-of-war for Lady Castleton upon her death.

Staking these claims to Lady Castleton can seem a curious twist on seventeenth-century colonial impulses, with the land itself declaring sovereignty over its inhabitants, yet this rhetoric highlights a strand of medical thought regarding bodies and their physical surroundings that was increasingly put to trial. Early modern physicians like William Bullein repeated Hippocratic notions that the climate into which individuals were born determined where they would thrive and where they might suffer.[4] As Andrew Wear puts it, the Hippocratic *Airs, Waters, Places* tradition's assertion that "the body was made up of the same qualities as climate" forged an essential link "between people, places, and health."[5] It then follows that ingredients and practices reflecting a person's geographical home would prove more suited to their care. For Timothie Bright and George Herbert,

2 Paula Watson and Paul Gauci, "George, 5th Visct. Castleton [I] (1631–1714), of Sandbeck, Yorks," in *The History of Parliament: The House of Commons 1690–1715*, eds. D. Hayton, E. Cruickshanks, and S. Handley (London: Boydell and Brewer, 2002).

3 Sh., *A Funeral Elegy*, 1.

4 William Bullein, *The Government of Health* (London, 1595), 29–31.

5 Andrew Wear, "Place, Health, and Disease: The Airs, Waters, Places Tradition in Early Modern England and North America," *Journal of Medieval and Early Modern Studies* 38, no. 3 (2008): 461.

the connection held so much power that using local herbs even takes on spiritual dimensions.[6]

As Gitanjali Shahani and Wendy Wall point out, the enormously popular author Gervase Markham emphasized to his early modern readers that the proper English housewife should use foods and medicines derived "more from the prouision of her owne yarde, than the furniture of the markets."[7] Such strictures, Shahani points out, meant that women could be blamed for allowing potentially damaging influences from abroad to find their way into their domestic domains. Since decisions about what a household consumed were overseen by women, they could be held responsible for exposing family members to humorally unsuitable, and therefore physically corrupting, forces. This power to "somehow 'English' foreign ingredients" left women responsible for the effects that these imports might have on the bodies they medicated and fed.[8] Physicians like Bright condemned the "over hastie use of such strange Merchandise" when instead English households should turn "to those wee knowe both in the blade, and in the seede, in the roote, & in the fruit, & know the aire, the hill, the valley, the medowe or Marsh ground where they growe."[9] Local botanical sources were simply superior to those from abroad, because they grew from familiar earth and breathed the same air as the patients they treated.[10] As the puritan physician Thomas Tryon argued almost a century later, "[O]ur *Fore-Fathers* lived not only as well, but

6 See Madeline Bassnett, *Women, Food Exchange, and Governance in Early Modern England* (New York: Palgrave Macmillan, 2016), 111–12. See also Mary Floyd-Wilson's notion of geo-humoralism as outlined in "English Mettle," in *Reading the Early Modern Passions: Essays in the Cultural History of Emotion*, eds. Gail Kern Paster, Katherine Rowe, and Mary Floyd-Wilson (Philadelphia: University of Pennsylvania Press, 2004), 130–46.

7 Gervase Markham, *Countrey Contentments, or The English Husvvife* (London, 1615), 4. This passage has garnered a great deal of attention, notably from Kim F. Hall, "Culinary Spaces, Colonial Spaces: The Gendering of Sugar in the Seventeenth Century," in *Feminist Readings of Early Modern Culture: Emerging Subjects*, eds. Valerie Traub and M. Lindsay Kaplan (Cambridge: University of Cambridge, 1996), 182; Gitanjali G. Shahani, *Tasting Difference: Food, Race, and Cultural Encounters in Early Modern Literature* (Ithaca: Cornell University Press, 2020), 24; and Wendy Wall, *Staging Domesticity: Household Work and English Identity in Early Modern Drama* (Cambridge: Cambridge University Press, 2002), 39–41.

8 Shahani, *Tasting Difference*, 34.

9 Timothie Bright, *A Treatise, vvherein is Declared the Sufficiencie of English Medicines* (London, 1615), 13.

10 This might also factor into concerns about the quality of imported goods, which, as Shahani points out, often suffered because of the lack of knowledge, and downright dishonesty, of the merchants who dealt in these materials. She points out that Hannah Woolley blames merchants for the bad quality of imported ingredients, which linger in storage "so long before they come to our hands, that they have lost half their virtue." See Shahani, *Tasting Difference*, 39 and Woolley, *The Gentlewomans Companion* (London, 1673), 165.

much better too" before imported ingredients like sugar and tobacco were readily available. The English, he claims, "were stronger, lustier, longer-liv'd and freed from Diseases, before the use of such things, than their Posterity are since; nay, many Diseases which we now-a-days groan under, were not then known."[11] But both Tryon and Bright realize that some imported ingredients would be used, regardless of these protests; in such cases, the practitioner should temper the unfamiliar humors of these imports to make them less shocking to the English system. Tryon, for example, argues that imported raisins can be beneficial so long as they are eaten alongside (but not baked into) bread.

Even more remarkably, Bright figures the English climate as the ultimate judge of a plant's suitability for English medicines. Furthering his assertion that medicinal herbs should be grown locally, Bright points out that imported plants can be nurtured quite successfully in magically fertile English ground:

> Our English soyle is greatly commended, as it iustly deserveth, for temper of the aire: & of such as have experience thereof, or strangers, and great masters of simples, for varietie of excellent medicines carrieth great praise, who report they finde such simples in the valleys and woodes of our North parts, as they finde in the toppes of mountaines in the South countries. So that certaine gardines in England, especially in London, are able to affourd great varietie of medicines even of forraine simples to all diseases.[12]

Even if they have origins abroad, plants that can thrive in England are just a little less foreign. Embedded in Bright's comments, however, is a concession to biodiversity within England. London's gardens no doubt "affourd great varietie" because more imported plants landed there, and because medical organizations like the College of Physicians and the Company of Barber Surgeons sponsored their cultivation. The "valleys and woodes of our North parts," however, sprout plants with these curative properties on their own, in a way not characteristic of other parts of England. The soil in places like Yorkshire, that is, can be commended on different terms than that in places elsewhere in England.

As Bright's comments suggest, medical materials traveled within England as well as into the country from overseas, with rural practices and ingredients, as well as bodies, making their way to English cities and vice versa.

11 Thomas Tryon, *The Good House-wife Made a Doctor* (London, 1692), 144.

12 Bright, *A Treatise*, 61–62.

This migration obscured local authority and regional knowledge, and also corresponded with the increasingly prevalent, seeming contradictory, idea among practitioners that the human body was perhaps more of a uniform construction than humoral theory imagined.[13] Tryon, for example, reveals during a reverie about the robust bodies of country women that they are in fact biologically the same as those of pampered city-dwelling "*good Dames*" who have allowed foreign goods and even warm clothing to alter their constitution. Addressing these privileged women, he asks:

> Are you, I say, with all this Furniture free from *catching Cold*, any more than the *Rosie-Complexion'd Lass* that courts the sweet kisses of the Air in her *Smock Sleeves*, and trips over the *Dewy-Plains* in a *Winters Frosty Morning* with but a *brace* of *Linsey-Woosley Coats* that are not long enough to conceal the shape of her *Well-Proportioned Legg*?[14]

Clearly, he can picture his more urbane female readers running, lightly clad, through the damp fields just as easily as country women, flashing identically attractive ankles. According to this logic, whether from the North or the South of England, bodies native to the island country resembled one another more than they differed. This, despite Tryon's insistence that Londoners are further removed from the purer, simpler country diets of bread and cheese that in "former Ages, when Sugar *Spanish* Fruits, Spices, Sweet Meats, and the like were not known in these Northern Climates."[15]

When apothecaries put local herbs and imported animal products side by side in their shops, these goods from vastly different locations transformed into a common *materia medica*, supposedly equally beneficial to all. As Whyte, van der Geest, and Hardon point out, these medical products are also "the most personal of material objects, swallowed, inserted into bodies, rubbed on by anxious mothers, used to express care and intimately empower the uncertain individual."[16] The cures Lady Castleton compiles make clear

13 Harold J. Cook for one argues that the notion that "all people possessed a common biology" rather than a quirky individualized humoral balance "was given a strong push from the development of a consumer market for medicines that would have similar effects on anyone who used them." See Harold J. Cook, "Markets and Cultures: Medical Specifics and the Reconfiguration of the Body in Early Modern Europe," *Transactions of the Royal Historical Society* 21 (2011): 130, 144.

14 Tryon, *The Good House-wife Made a Doctor*, 108.

15 Tryon, *The Good House-wife Made a Doctor*, 86. See Hall, "Culinary Spaces, Colonial Spaces" for a discussion of Tryon's racially charged discussion of the inhabitants of East India and the Americas and the impact of their products on English bodies.

16 Susan Reynolds Whyte, et al., *The Social Lives of Medicine* (Cambridge: Cambridge University Press, 2002), 3.

that the tensions associated with the medical marketplace not only permeated domestic practice, but had long influenced rural healthcare in parts of England far outside metropolitan centers. Her manuscript illustrates how recipes for home-based treatments absorb and reject changes in practice as they travel through social and commercial networks, encompassing both rural and urban knowledge, before going on to transform the bodies of those making and taking the treatments produced.

The Family Roots of Lady Grace Castleton's Manuscript

Folger MS V.a. 600, the recipe compilation that Grace Belasyse Saunderson, Lady Castleton initiated, offers a vivid glimpse of her experience of her surroundings, allowing us to see her as manipulating her environment rather than simply blending into it.[17] The compilation reflects the Yorkshire towns and family connections that surrounded her before her marriage, though other, further flung locales make their presence known in her recipes as well. In fact, Lady Castleton's recipes reveal that her kin had assimilated some foreign materials into the family's practices well before her birth in 1635. Grace grew up a member of the Belasyse family, the most affluent family in the North Riding of Yorkshire.[18] Their estate at Newburgh Priory offered ready access to native medicinal plants, thanks to its situation near a spot on the parish map called "Farmacy Hill" (figure 1).[19] Her recipe manuscript is clearly labeled with her husband's name, suggesting that she began keeping the book around the time of her marriage to George Saunderson, Viscount Castleton, of Saxby, Lincolnshire in 1656. While Saunderson owned estates in both Yorkshire and Lincolnshire, Lady Castleton seems to have kept close to her roots at Newburgh Priory. The couple's children were born at Sandbeck Park, not more than thirty miles from her girlhood Yorkshire home, and at least one child was baptized in the same parish, Coxwold, where Lady Castleton herself had been christened.[20]

17 Lady Grace Castleton, *The Lady Grace Castleton's Booke of Receipts*, seventeenth century, Folger MS V.a. 600, Folger Shakespeare Library, Washington, DC.

18 The Newburgh Priory estate was valued at £4000 per year in 1611; in 1624, its total value was estimated as £8000. See J.T. Cliffe, *The Yorkshire Gentry from the Reformation to the Civil War* (London: Athlone Press, 1969), 110–11. In 1609, the estate employed fifty-one servants. See Cliffe, *The Yorkshire Gentry*, 113.

19 See Francis Mayson, *A Plat of theise Lordships Videlicet Newebrough, Cockewolde, Owleston, Yearsley*, 1605, North Yorkshire County Council County Records Office.

20 The Coxwold parish registries note her first son's birth as follows: "George Sanderson sonne and Heire to the right Honourable George Lord Vicount Castlton borne 10 Sep 1654 in the Yeare

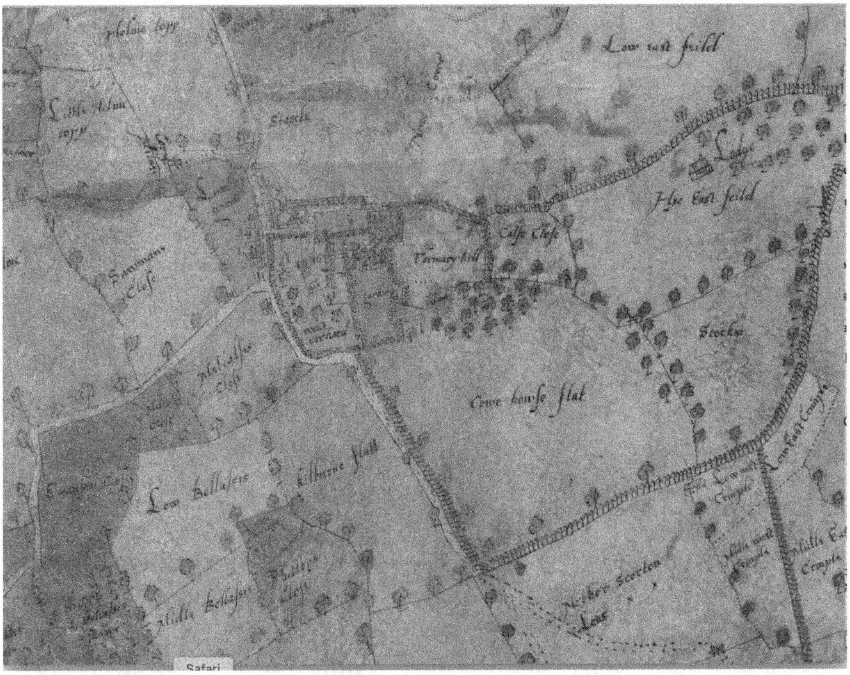

Figure 1. Farmacy Hill, a source for medicinal plants located near properties owned by the Belasyse family in Yorkshire. From Francis Mayson, *A Plat of theise Lordships Videlicet Newebrough, Cockewolde, Owleston, Yearsley*, 1605. Courtesy of the North Yorkshire County Council County Records Office.

Lady Castleton kept her recipe book for just over ten years, beginning in 1656 and using it until her death in London in 1667.[21] This said, it would be an oversimplification to see these years as the firm starting and ending dates for Lady Castleton's portion of the manuscript, because, like all manuscript recipe collections, it reaches both forward and backward in time in unannounced ways. Some of collection's recipes existed well before Lady Castleton began her book; her death, moreover, did not end the manuscript, which made its way to a second owner. This makes clear

of our Lord God." Her own birth is recorded in the same registry, as "Gracia Belassis filia Henrici de Oulstone armigeri bapt.est 14 May 1635." See M. F. Wilson, *Coxwold parish register transcripts 1583–1666*, https://archive.org/details/CoxwoldParishRegisterTranscripts1583–1666, accessed February 3, 2021.

21 How often she journeyed between London and Yorkshire in these years is not clear. As Leong has shown, women leaving the country for London could remain deeply involved in the affairs of their rural homes, ordering servants to make and send to the city medicines more easily produced in the country, while sending imports home. See Elaine Leong, *Recipes and Everyday Knowledge* (Chicago: University of Chicago Press, 2018), 46–70.

a fundamental principle of early modern recipe manuscripts: it is nearly impossible to examine fairly just one recipe, or one recipe book, because these texts are always embedded in a complex web of family relationships and environmental influences. Rather than see these recipes preserving practices as they preserve, say, apricots, it is more accurate to see them as starting points for envisioning medicines and ingredients as parts of knowledge networks permeating different environments, where they might be renamed and used for different purposes. And, as we shall see, recipes manifested in this particular manuscript land differently—sometimes drastically changed and sometimes barely modified—when they appear in different collections.

This manuscript luckily offers a partial record of its own historical connections, hinting at links to a second compilation. Lady Grace Castleton attributes five recipes in her pages of V.a. 600 to a "Lady Lister," whose mention in the funeral elegy suggests that she might be a significant force in Lady Castleton's life (the poet remarks "Her dear Aunt Lister (whom she lov'd) and she, / How well in Heav'n now do they agree?"). Mary Belasyse, sister of Lady Grace Castleton's grandfather Thomas Belasyse, 1st Lord Fauconberg of Yarm, married Sir William Lister in 1610. Fortunately, the University of Leeds counts among its early modern recipe manuscripts a *Recipe Book Known as "Dame Mary Lister's Household Book"*, with the years 1625–35 stamped in gold on its front cover.[22] Yet not a single one of the recipes Lady Grace Castleton attributes in her book to Lady Lister appears in this manuscript—which may suggest that Lady Lister kept an additional recipe collection. But Lady Lister's manuscript contains something even more enticing: a section of recipes attributed to Grace Belasyse, Lady Grace Castleton's mother.[23] These thirteen recipes are linked by a common hand, distinct from the book's other handwriting, and one cure "For a consumtion" proclaims itself as "tried by mee G:B." The treatment is also labeled as reflecting "Mr. Doctor Butler['s] advice," but G.B's—that is, Grace Belasyse's—probatum takes equal weight, if not precedence, in the recipe title. Even more striking: Lady Grace Castleton includes this same recipe in her book, without mention of either her mother or her great aunt, even though she seems to have had

22 Mary Lister, *Recipe Book Known as "Dame Mary Lister's Household Book,"* 1625–35, University of Leeds MS 621, University of Leeds, Leeds, England.

23 Lady Castleton and her mother share the name Grace; I have used fuller versions of their names in this paragraph in hopes of setting out the genealogy clearly. Smith provides a helpful family tree showing these relationships on the back flyleaf of *In Well Beware*. See Geoffrey Ridsill Smith, *In Well Beware: The Story of Newburgh Priory and the Belsayse Family, 1145–1977* (Kineton: Roundwood Press, 1978).

either her mother's or Lady Lister's book nearby as she copied this recipe; in fact, it could be that Grace Belasyse took Lady Lister's book as her own, adding recipes after Mary's death in 1653.

Rather than name her great aunt or her mother as local authorities endorsing her copied cure for consumption, Lady Castleton notes the origin as Doctor Butler, a person whom she may never have met but whose title signals his endorsement by the wider, professional healthcare establishment.[24] Indeed, Dr. William Butler was a well-known Cambridge doctor and member of the London College of Physicians whose name was often invoked in recipe manuscripts.[25] Medical authority obscures family connections, at least where the written rather than the memorial record is concerned.

For a consumtion by D. Buttler.	For a Consumption Mr. Doctor Butler advice And tried by mee G:B
Take an ould cock sume 2 or 3 yeare ould dray him & dress him but [put] him stons & come & all into a pipkin with a gallon of fare runing water & boyle him well on a charcole fire & when the skim rises take it of & then put into the pipkin 2 ouncis of cheany cutt small & one handfull of made= ons haire & one handfull of white Arck= angell & one pound of rasons of the sonn	Take an old Cocke some two or three yeare olde or older if you can gett him. Draw him and quarter him, and put him, combe stones, and all into a fayre earthen pott. with a gallon of fayre run inge water, and boyle him well, on chare coole fire, and when the skim rise, take itt off, and then putt it into the pott two ounces of cheanye, cut small: and one handfull of maydene hayre, and one handfull of white Arke

24 On the likely lack of connection between manuscript owners and the authorities they cite, see Michelle DiMeo, "Authorship and Medical Networks," in *Reading and Writing Recipe Books, 1550–1800*, eds. Michelle DiMeo and Sara Pennell (Manchester: Manchester University Press, 2013), 25–46.

25 See Margaret Pelling and Frances White, "BUTLER, William," in *Physicians and Irregular Medical Practitioners in London 1550–1640 Database* (London: Centre for Metropolitan History, 2004), *British History Online*, and Matthew Butler, "William Butler (1535–1618): A Biography of a Singular Physician," *Journal of Medical Biography* 1 (2023): 1–8. A Granville family manuscript offers a version as "Doctor Butlers Receipt against a consumption," and Rawdon labels a similar concoction in his manuscript recipes book as "sett downe by docter | Buttler of Cambridge"; both incorporate China root and omit the gold. See Granville Family, *Cookery and Medical Receipts of the Granville Family, c. 1640–c. 1750*, Folger MS V.a. 430, Folger Shakespeare Library, Washington, DC, 49, also transcribed in Kristine Kowalchuk, *Preserving on Paper: Seventeenth-Century Englishwoman's Receipt Books* (Toronto: University of Toronto Press, 2017), 92–93, as well as Marmaduke Rawdon, *Medical Receipts*, 1637, University of Minnesota MS WZ250 M489, Owen H. Wangensteen Historical Library of Biology and Medicine, Minneapolis, MN, 197. Lady Ayscough offers a recipe in her manuscript for "Buttler Generall Dyatt drink," also featuring China root, which also repeats the name "Dr. Buttler" at the end. See Lady Ayscough, *Receits of Phisick and Chirurgery*, 1692, Wellcome MS 1026, Wellcome Collection, London, England, 220–21.

stoned & one pound of dat[e]s stoned, one ounce of harts horne & x peices of ould gould lett all these boyle in it 6 houers then take it of & strene it well, this broth will, Ielly & you must take 4 sponfulls in a morn= ing & the same quanity in the after noune soe long as it lasteth	Angell, and one pound of raysons of the Sunn stoned, and one pund of dates stoned, one ounce of harts horne, and ten peeces of olde gouled let all these things boyle in it five hours, then take it of and straine it well, till there be noo juce in the Cocke. This Brothe will jelley, and you must take foure spoonfulls in a morning, and the same quantitie in the after no one soo long as it lastesth.
–*The Lady Grace Castleton's Booke of Receipts*[26]	–*Recipe Book Known as "Dame Mary Lister's Household Book"*[27]

Lady Castleton's care in retaining this record of outside authority appears even more remarkable given the homely nature of most of the ingredients in "For a consumtion." It is, in essence, a chicken broth with herbs, something that to modern sensibilities aligns with domestic cures rather than those formally prescribed by doctors.[28] The "x peices of ould gould" stand out as an unexpected, unhomely ingredient, though even that rare component has a long history in fever and plague cures.[29]

But this otherwise straightforward broth does require an ingredient only recently available in England: China root, or "cheany." Used initially among Europeans to fight syphilis, China root became immensely valued in other medical contexts as well, ranking among the top five drugs imported into England as pharmaceutical trade expanded between 1567 and 1774.[30] The result is a supercharged curative masquerading as a humble broth, one that incorporates newer ingredients into a proven formula to reflect

26 Castleton, *The Lady Grace Castleton's Booke of Receipts*, seventeenth century, Folger MS V.a. 600, 39.

27 Lister, *Recipe Book Known as "Dame Mary Lister's Household Book,"* 1625–35, University of Leeds MS 621, 55.

28 This corresponds with Anne Stobart's conclusions in her exhaustive examination of ingredients in early modern recipe manuscripts, where she found that in the seventeenth century "there was potential for sourcing almost 27 per cent of recipe ingredients from the garden, with the remaining ingredients split between household (3.7 per cent), kitchen (13.3 per cent), apothecary (38.4 per cent) and the wild (16.9 per cent)." See Anne Stobart, *Household Medicine in Seventeenth-Century England* (London: Bloomsbury, 2016), 83.

29 Renzo Console, "Pharmaceutical Use of Gold from Antiquity to the Seventeenth Century," in *A History of Geology in Medicine*, eds. C. Duffin, R. T. J. Moody, and C. Gardner-Thorpe (London: Geological Society of London, 2013), 171–91.

30 Patrick Wallis, "Exotic Drugs and English Medicine: England's Drug Trade, c. 1550–c. 1800," *Social History of Medicine* 25, no. 1 (2012): 20–46 and Anna E. Winterbottom, "Of the China Root: A Case Study of the Early Modern Circulation of Materia Medica," *Social History of Medicine* 28, no. 1 (2014): 22–44.

cutting-edge knowledge.[31] Where the Belasyse family would have gotten their China root is unclear, but records suggest several possible routes for the arrival of imported botanicals into Yorkshire. P. M. Stell notes that ten apothecaries operated in the medieval city of York in the fifteenth century, one of whom ordered stock from Flanders, to be imported through Hull, while other city apothecaries relied on London for their supplies.[32] In 1617, Henry Best mentions bringing home to Yorkshire an array of medical ingredients, ranging from spices like ginger, cloves, and pepper; to prepared rosewater and aquavitae; to the especially exotic bezor stone and ambergris. Unfortunately, he does not say where he bought them. Best does offer a sketch of local fairs, though, noting that the Beverly fair in May is particularly well-stocked since "thither the Londoners sende their wares by water, and thither come the Yorke grocers and others."[33] While drugs and treatments often flowed from London to the north, Linda Levy Peck adds that Yorkshire families sent their sons as apprentices to the Grocers and Apothecaries companies in London, building both knowledge and pharmaceutical networks in the process.[34]

Making Green Ointment in Yorkshire

While the adherence to her mother's recipe might suggest that Lady Castleton tends to simply repeat received knowledge, her recipe "To make the grene ointment" recognizes and assesses her predecessors' experimentation. She studies her local sources, that is, before committing to her own version. Her green ointment seems at first to be a close copy of her mother's—again, as it is recorded in Lady Lister's book.

31 Versions of this gold-infused broth appeared in print, too, often among culinary recipes; Hannah Woolley's chicken broth with gold and China root, for example, appears under the title "To make a Cordial strength|ning Broath" and is directly followed by "To Candy Grapes." See Hannah Woolley, *The Accomplish'd Lady's Delight* (London, 1675), 77–78.

32 See P. M. Stell, "The Apothecaries of Medieval York," *York Historian* 14 (1976): 26–31 and Patrick Wallis, "Apothecaries and the Consumption and Retailing of Medicines in Early Modern London," in *From Physick to Pharmacology: Five Hundred Years of British Drug Retailing*, ed., Louise Hill Curth (London: Routledge, 2016), 17–18. For more on the role grocers played in this process, see Jon Stobart, *Sugar and Spice: Grocers and Groceries in Provincial England, 1650–1830* (Oxford: Oxford University Press, 2013).

33 See Henry Best, *Rural Economy in Yorkshire in 1641, being the Farm and Account Books of Henry Best*, ed. Charles Best Robinson (Durham: Publications of the Surtees Society, 1857), 150, 112.

34 See Linda Levy Peck, *Women of Fortune: Money, Marriage, and Murder in Early Modern England* (Cambridge: Cambridge University Press, 2018), 45–72.

To make the grene oyntment	To make the greene oyntment
Take red sage leavs & rue of each a pound the youngest bay Leaus & wormwood of each halfe a pound pick them wach them & cut them small & bray them lone in a fare morter then take 3 pound of sheep lever [suet] hot from the sheepe minch it small & beat it with those hearbs till all be of the coler then put all into a fare bottel bowell of the best oyle olive working all together till it be a littill soft put it then into an earthen pott stop it close after 7 days then boyle all together on a swelt fire put to it when it is halfe boyled 4 ouncis of oyle of spich …	Take red sage and rue of each a quarte the youngest bay leaves and woorme wood of each halph a pound picke them, wash them and cutt them small, and braye them longe in a fayer morter, then take five pound of sheepe suet, hott from the sheepe, mash itt smale, and beat it with those hearbs till all be of one culler, then put all into a fayre pottle bowle, of the best oyle olive, workinge all together till itt be a little soft. putt it then int an earthen pott stop it close for 8 or 9 dayes then seeth all together in a fayre pan on a soft fire, put to it halph sodden 3 ounces of oyle of spetch …
–*The Lady Grace Castleton's Booke of Receipts*[35]	–*Recipe Book known as "Dame Mary Lister's Household Book"*[36]

These recipes certainly echo one another, but it is important to note that Lady Castleton's version consults two versions of the recipe preserved in Lady Lister's manuscript. The green ointment recipe is repeated later in Lady Lister's collection, in a different hand than the version cited above, with some slight but telling variations. This second version in turn seeps into Lady Castleton's rendition of the recipe. Though it describes the same ingredients and proportions, this second version suggests keeping the concoction in earthen pots for "6 days in the Sonne" and carries an attribution noting "this has been tride by William Coocke." The second version also offers more details regarding the ointment's use, specifying "the bigness of ahalfe a | pea of this ointments chafed into the sore & | stoped with blacke wool, helpeth all pains."[37] These adjustments suggest Lady Castleton considered and conflated the two versions set down in Lady Lister's collection to make a single entry. Not only does Lady Castleton's version compromise on the storage time—averaging the advice to let the mixture sit for "6 days" or "8 or 9" days to settle on 7—she offers a follow-up to explain "the virtues" of the

35 Castleton, *The Lady Grace Castleton's Booke of Receipts*, Folger MS V.a. 600, 18–19.

36 Lister, *Recipe Book Known as "Dame Mary Lister's Household Book,"* University of Leeds MS 621, 62.

37 Lister, *Recipe Book Known as "Dame Mary Lister's Household Book,"* University of Leeds MS 621, 67.

ointment in helping digestion, backaches, and the stone before concluding that "stored close with blackwool [it] helpeth all pean [pain]."[38] The specification of the black wool appears only in the recipe's second manifestation in Lady Lister's book, suggesting that Lady Castleton integrated it into her more thorough, though certainly not authoritative, single manuscript entry. The Belasyse family, after all, did not invent green ointments, and variations on this cure appear in texts dating before and after their books.[39] In fact, Lady Castleton's omission of William Coocke's name may reflect an awareness that the recipe itself is common, if not communal, something that can be traced only to the place where it was learned.

All of the Castleton-related green ointment recipes reflect a rural location, bringing local ingredients, specifically those derived from sheep, into the care of local bodies in a way that not all green ointment recipes do. Requiring suet be "hot from the sheepe," Lady Lister's and Lady Castleton's green ointments assume immediate access to livestock, something easier to achieve in the country than in London. Several other recipe manuscripts with Yorkshire connections require suet "hot" from the sheep for green ointments as well.[40] Evoking without detailing this scene of butchery, these recipes insert a small space between recipe makers and the actual killing of the animal.[41] Nonetheless, making these Yorkshire green ointment recipes requires intense work with many parts of the sheep carcass. The "oyl of spich"—also known as "spetch grease"—indicated a second sheep product, derived from soaking its leather in water to create "an oylie grease."[42] And, of course, black wool would be nearby during these processes as well. Prepared as directed, with

38 Castleton, *The Lady Grace Castleton's Booke of Receipts*, Folger MS V.a. 600, 19.

39 Lady Lister actually has a third green ointment much later in her book, involving sallet oil as well as sheep suet. It also makes no mention of black wool. See Lister, *Recipe Book Known as "Dame Mary Lister's Household Book,"* University of Leeds MS 621, 147.

40 Lady Ayscough's Yorkshire-connected recipe book requires "hot" sheep suet in its green ointment, as do two manuscripts associated with the Fairfax family—also in Yorkshire. See Ayscough, *Receipts of Phisick and Chirurgery*, 1692, Wellcome MS 1026, 14; Elizabeth Fairfax, *Manuscript Book of Culinary and Medicinal Recipes in Several Hands*, 1694, GMU C0202, George Mason University, Fairfax, VA, 123; and *Arcana Fairfaxiana Manuscripta*, ed. G. Weddell, 64. A very similar recipe appears in Jane Randolph's Virginia manuscript, dated 1743 and treated in chapter 4, only there it is titled "For make Dr Butlers Oyl"; it calls for "Seuet hot out of [th]e Sheep." See Katherine E. Harbury, *Colonial Virginia's Cooking Dynasty* (Columbia: University of South Carolina Press, 2004), 330.

41 Fairfax makes explicit mention of a sheep butcher, including a smallpox treatment that asks for "12 sheepps treekless newly made or gitt a quan|tity from the Buchter that kills a sheep." See Fairfax, *Manuscript Book of Culinary and Medicinal Recipes in Several Hands*, 1694, GMU MS C0202, 117.

42 "spetch, n.," in *Oxford English Dictionary*, July 18, 2023. Some green ointment recipes require "oil of spike," perhaps as a result of regional misunderstanding, copying error, or purposeful

local herbs and leaves, the result is an ointment made of Yorkshire plants and animals for use on bodies firmly connected to the same land.

Similar green ointments, however, appear in the less geographically rooted realm of professional medicine, where bodies were increasingly seen as responding uniformly to treatments regardless of their humoral balances. A green ointment, for example, appears alongside handwritten transcriptions of lectures offered at the Worshipful Society of Apothecaries of London in a 1634 notebook. Labeled as a "Pretious Greene Oynment," the recipe requires "sheepes suet pickt cleane from the skynn," but it makes no demands that it be "hot."[43] Popular guidebooks like *The Queen's Closet Opened* include green ointment recipes that contain similar ingredients,[44] and the overwhelming majority take their sheep suet at whatever temperature and freshness they can get it, perhaps because it is only available separate from the animal. One notable exception: *Natura Exenterata*, a printed collection of recipes culled from women's manuscript compilations, contains three recipes for three different green ointments, and one, by Lady Constable (of Benton Constable, East Yorkshire), requires suet "hot from the sheep."[45]

Seasonality and Green Ointment, Further Afield

As consistent as these seemingly rural ingredients—and perhaps origins—for green ointment appear, and even if they are indeed trustworthy glimpses

adjustment. Anne Stobart includes one such recipe, from Lady Clifford's 1690 manuscript. See Stobart, *Household Medicine in Seventeenth-Century England*, 43.

43 Worshipful Society of the Apothecaries of London, *Medical miscellany* [manuscript], ca. 1634, Folger MS E.a.5, Folger Shakespeare Library, Washington, DC, 113r. For an examination of the manuscript, see Dmitri Levitin, "'Made Up from Many Experimentall Notions': The Society of Apothecaries, Medical Humanism, and the Rhetoric of Experience in 1630s London," *Journal of British* Studies 21, no. 2 (1982): 549–87.

44 *The Queens Closet Opened* (London, 1659), 97.

45 Philiatros, *Natura Exenterata: or Nature Unbowelled* (London: 1655), 250. Spiller connects Philatros to Aletheia Talbot, whose picture appears at the opening of *Natura Exenterata*; see Elizabeth Spiller, *Seventeenth-Century English Recipe Books: Cooking, Physic and Chirurgery in the Works of Elizabeth Talbot Grey and Aletheia Talbot Howard* (Burlington: Ashgate, 2011). In her discussion of Ann Fanshawe, Lucy Moore notes that Brilliana Harley also had a green ointment recipe in her manuscript recipe book, BL Egerton MS2214. See Lucy Moore, *Lady Fanshawe's Receipt Book: The Life and Times of a Civil War Heroine* (London: Atlantic, 2017), 54. Not all recipes for green ointments, it is important to note, contain suet. Chantrell, for example, uses butter; see Mary Chantrell, *Book of Receipts*, 1690, Wellcome MS.1548, Wellcome Collection, London, England, 30r. For a discussion of this recipe, see Susan H. Brandt, *Women Healers: Gender, Authority, and Medicine in Early Philadelphia* (Philadelphia: University of Pennsylvania Press, 2022), 26.

into pastoral roots, the mobility of the recipe constantly widens the gap between home medical practice and the rural fields it evokes. Two examples of the medicine's appearance outside of Yorkshire offer vivid proof that this green ointment, with suet "hot from the sheep" and all, earned popularity in a wider geographical area. It is possible that Lady Castleton may well have played a role in this, passing the recipe to other nonlocal compilers during her time in London, though no evidence of such an uncomplicated chain of transmission presents itself—and in fact, the hazy dating of at least one of these manuscripts render that path extremely unlikely.

Lady Katherine Sandys is the implied source of a green ointment recipe recorded in a seventeenth-century manuscript held at Princeton University's Firestone library. After copying more than ninety recipes, the book's early seventeenth-century compiler marks out a new section, declaring "Hear begins my Lady | Sandys her receipts." This notation has led scholars to connect the volume to the family of Sir Edwin Sandys, specifically to his wife Katherine Bulkeley Sandys whom he married in 1605. Neither Katherine, who survived until 1634, nor the Sandys family originated in Yorkshire, but Sir Edwin Sandys inherited land holdings there from his father, Edwin Sandys, Archbishop of York; these lands were substantial enough to generate revenue that supported Katherine after her husband's death.[46] It is tempting to imagine that those connections account for the compiler's inclusion of a recipe for "The green oyntment good for aches, scabs, | fellons, anguish or swelling, toothach, bruises, | over straining of the sinnews, pains, cramps, | stiches, scyatica, burnings, scaldings, stifle, | strain, or swelling, to be made in may only."[47] The ingredients, proportions, and procedures—including the hot suet—are identical to those Lady Lister and Lady Castleton recorded. In fact, given the vagaries of establishing dates for these collections, it is quite possible that the Sandys manuscript's version was recorded even before the Yorkshire compilers committed their surviving versions to paper, in 1625 at the earliest.[48] An attribution to "Aunt Frances" accompanies the Sandys recipe,[49] and she, like

46 See Theodore K. Rabb, "Sandys, Sir Edwin (1561–1629), Politician and Colonial Entrepreneur," in *Oxford Dictionary of National Biography*, September 23, 2004, accessed July 18, 2023 and Patrick Collinson, "Sandys, Edwin (1519?–1588), archbishop of York," in *Oxford Dictionary of National Biography*, September 23, 2004, accessed October 13, 2024. Catherine's family originated in Wales, and she and Edwin spent most of their married life in London and Kent.

47 *English Receipt Book*, seventeenth century, Princeton MS RTC01 no. 208, Princeton University, Princeton, NJ, 63v.

48 Lady Lister's manuscript is dated 1625, though its recipes may predate that designation. Edwin Sandys's first wife died by 1588, if the Lady Sandys named is indeed the wife of Edwin.

49 The Princeton University catalog record suggests "Aunt Frances" could be the sister of the Edwin's father (1519–1585). See https://catalog.princeton.edu/catalog/9940049493506421. Rabb

many named sources, remains unidentified. The Sandys collection, however, puts this green ointment recipe in a remarkably new context, situating it among cures that reflect the family's connections to lands across the Atlantic. As we shall see, Edwin Sandys was deeply involved in the Virginia Company, investing in 1606 and serving as treasurer by 1619, though he never left England to tend to related duties. Neither did Katherine, but her recipes incorporate American ingredients such as tobacco, sassafras, and, yes, China root.[50]

Lady Grace Carteret, 1st Countess Granville, whose manuscript begins a generation or so after Lady Castleton's, also offers a nearly identical green ointment recipe despite her different geographical roots. She was heir to her father's estates in Cornwall and Bath, far from the northern counties Lady Castleton knew. Her husband's family connections, however, exerted a significant influence on her recipe collection, which shares many entries with the book compiled by Lady Ann Fanshawe. Fanshawe's connection to the Carteret family predated Grace's marriage into it, perhaps even predating Grace's birth; significant parts of the families' bond, moreover, took root as Fanshawe stayed at the Carteret home in Jersey while in the process of fleeing the country during the Civil War. The Fanshawes even left their young daughter with Elizabeth, an earlier Lady Carteret, during their travels when exiled.[51] Thus, the later Lady Carteret's recipe books carry resonances of life in the Channel Islands even though she herself remained largely in London and on her own inherited estates. Her recipe for green ointment nonetheless echoes Castleton's assertion that the medicine, rolled into "the bignes of a small pea" and "put into the ear which stopped with black | wool," can "healpeth the paines thereof" and "tis to be made in | May only." She too still calls for "suet hot from the sheepe." Like Lady Sandys, she concludes that the ointment is good for "sciatica, | burns scarlds," before concluding that "tis to be made in | May only."[52]

only says that Frances "may well have been a relative of the compiler." See Theodore K. Rabb, "'My Lady Sandys her Receipts': A Manuscript of Cookery and Medicine," *The Princeton University Library Chronicle* 72, no. 2 (2011), 457.

50 See this book's epilogue.

51 See Ann Fanshawe, *The Memoirs of Ann, Lady Fanshawe*, in *The Memoirs of Anne, Lady Halkett and Ann, Lady Fanshawe*, ed. John Loftis (Oxford: Clarendon, 1979), 119, as well as the Carteret family tree in G. R. Balleine, *All for the King: The Life Story of Sir George Carteret* (St. Helier, Jersey: Société Jersiaise, 1976), 176–77. Helpful information on the family's generations appears in the biography of her son, John. See John Cannon, "Carteret, John, second Earl Granville (1690–1763), politician," in *Oxford Dictionary of National Biography*, September 23, 2004, accessed August 25, 2023.

52 Grace Carteret, *Manuscript Recipe book of Grace Carteret, 1st Countess Granville*, 1654–1744, Wellcome MS. 8903, Wellcome Collection, London, England, 77r.

Lady Sandys and Lady Carteret, in short, existed within networks with more immediate connections to further flung locations than Lady Castleton's three geographical points of contact named in the poem praising her. They nonetheless demand an immediacy between harvest and use, with their suet's temperature indicating a sheep's recent slaughter. Presumably, Carteret and Sandys could obtain fresh suet, either through access to their rural estates or at urban markets where freshly slaughtered sheep would likely be available for a premium price. But other ingredients—particularly sage and the required "youngest bay Leaus"—required harvesting at a particular time of the year, namely May. Lady Lister demands a May production date for green ointment, but she also is clearly assuming that the maker will be near the fields where the rue, sage, wormwood, and bay would be growing, since she directs her readers to "picke them" personally. The Sandys recipe makes a similar assumption, but Lady Carteret makes no references to picking at all. In her recipe, the herbs are strictly there for the taking—quite literally, since she uses the same exact verb, telling her reader to "Take redd sage and the rhue of each a pound, the youngest bay leaves, | wormewood of each halfe a pound, cutt & beat them well in a morter." She makes no requirement for picking the herbs, perhaps because she has no source for such immediate access. Whether in the islands, or in the city, her herbs may have come from local markets, grocers, or apothecaries. Yet she still insists the ointment is to be made "in May only."

Certainly, this emphasis on seasonality proves common among early modern recipe compilers. Jennifer Munroe argues that conscious attention to the rhythms of plant growth and availability suggest a keener connection between domestic production and the environment, while Elaine Leong shows that other recipe compilers, like Johanna St. John, saw seasonal availability as a challenge to be overcome.[53] Both underscore the predicaments that recipe requirements for the freshest herbs could pose. This insistence may not come from personal experience; it could simply be a direction copied from a source making explicit demands. In that case, recipes offer a veiled connection to other times and more rural places.

53 Jennifer Munroe, "Sympoeisis and Early Modern Cooking: Troubling the Boundaries of Human/Nonhuman," in *In the Kitchen, 1550–1800: Reading English Cooking at Home and Abroad,* eds. Madeline Bassnett and Hillary M. Nunn (Amsterdam: Amsterdam University Press), 29–44 and Leong, *Recipes and Everyday Knowledge*, 64–65. Wall's work with recipes as a mode of preserving perishable goods offers a valuable, food-centered look at seasonality as well. See Wendy Wall, *Recipes for Thought: Knowledge and Taste in the Early Modern Kitchen* (Philadelphia: University of Pennsylvania Press, 2015), 167–208.

But there could indeed be very valid reasons for retaining such demands far from a recipe's place of origin. Observations about weather conditions at the time of production could remain meaningful even when a recipe has migrated to a different location, but even more pertinent is the simple fact that markets too are subject to season. Just as produce available in grocery stores can reflect seasonal variation, the herbs available for purchase could do so as well. Thus, as much as these directions about seasonality can seem out of place, or even quaintly nostalgic, for recipes produced in the distant Jersey islands, or the cosmopolitan context of a London home, Lady Carteret's recipe reinscribes precautions that may well be vital to observe even in the surroundings where bay and wormwood are not easily gathered. This attention to seasonality sets the clock for these green ointment recipes, making clear that even the best early modern markets cannot evade the rhythms that climate and weather impose on the growth of herbs. But the ointment, on the other hand, can skirt these forces, combining its ingredients in such a way as to extend the temporal limitations of their effectiveness. As Lady Castleton puts it, the ointment is "only | made in may" but will "last | many years with carfull & coule setting."[54]

The recipes Lady Castleton records represent influences other than her family home, blending in ingredients from beyond Yorkshire even when she seems to be calling on local agricultural products; this reveals a dependence on local and international markets as well as on ingredients freely culled from her immediate surroundings. Her consumption recipe may look humble, but its requirement for gold challenges the resources of the English countryside. Even more telling, the plants and animal products that come together to make green ointment may vary, and suggest different forms of access to the sheep required to make it. While there are requirements about when the compound can be made, there are no recorded limits on where the medicine can be prepared, or used. The ointment makes no claims to curing everyone, but it rules no patients out as potential beneficiaries. Those with adequate access to its ingredients and to the knowledge needed

54 Castleton, *The Lady Grace Castleton's Booke of Receipts*, Folger MS V.a. 600, 20. Lady Constable echoes that sentiment in the more public forum of *Natura Exenterata* as well. Philiatros, *Natura Exenterata*, 250. The Constable family represented East Yorkshire ridings in Parliament throughout the seventeenth century. See David Scott, "Constable, Sir William, baronet (bap. 1590, d. 1655), Parliamentary army officer and Regicide," in *Oxford Dictionary of National Biography*, September 23, 2004, accessed August 28, 2003 and Simon Healy, "CONSTABLE, Sir Henry (1556/7–1607), or Burton Constable and Upsall Castle, Yorks," in *The History of Parliament: The House of Commons 1604–1629*, eds. Andrew Thrush and John P. Ferris (Cambridge: Cambridge University Press, 2010).

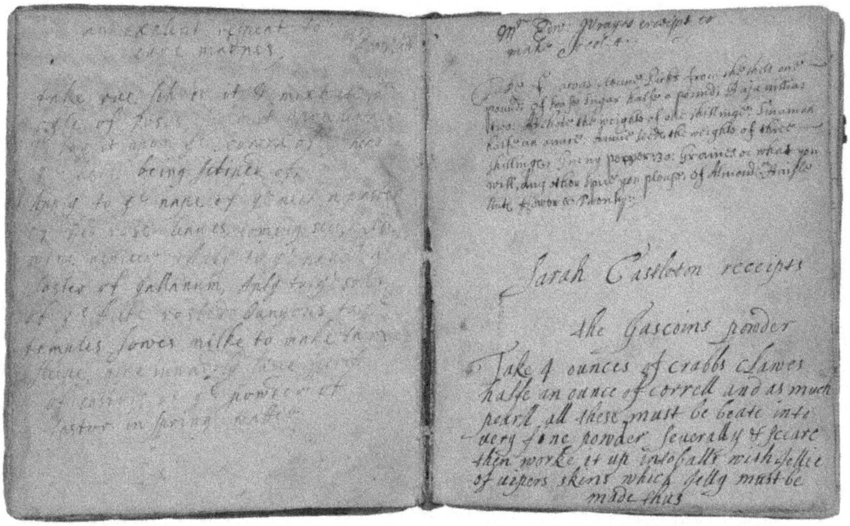

Figure 2. Sarah Fanshawe Saunderson, the new Lady Castleton, marks the transition to her recipes in the book she inherited from her predecessor, Lady Grace Castleton. From *The Lady Grace Castleton's Booke of Receipts,* seventeenth century, Folger MS V.a. 600, 124. Courtesy of the Folger Shakespeare Library.

to produce it are linked closely enough, in other words, to gain from its use. These patients may not have similar backgrounds, or in fact any connection to the neighboring lands, but their proximity to similar knowledge networks implies a fundamental physical similarity, despite preconceptions regarding humoral differences.

Just as the poetic tribute to Lady Castleton emphasizes the three different locations that could lay claim to her body, the recipe manuscript she kept owes a debt to forces beyond its first compiler for its vitality. The manuscript, after all, continued to grow after Lady Castleton's death, incorporating bits of other people's lives and knowledge at every step. The manuscript stayed with the Saunderson household, most likely because Lady Grace Castleton had no surviving daughter to take it with her to a new home. Instead, Saunderson's next wife, Lady Sarah, asserts her ownership of the manuscript with an audacious swirling signature in the book's center, in effect proclaiming not just the recipes that follow but the entire collection—and household—as her turf upon her marriage (figure 2).[55] Even more striking, the second Lady Castleton seems to have paid little attention to the recipes written down before her arrival, adding cures that repeat those already in the book. Her first addition to the manuscript echoes a cure from her aunt by marriage, the

55 Castleton, *The Lady Grace Castleton's Booke of Receipts*, Folger MS V.a. 600, 124.

renowned recipe collector Ann Fanshawe,[56] and one soon following looks back to Sarah's previous marriage to describe a cordial she made for her second husband. While she may have brought her own recipe book to the marriage, no record of one exists. Instead, the new Lady Castleton plunges herself into the household's existing book, writing herself into its history and geography, proclaiming herself—her past, as well as her present and future—to be perfectly at home in her new landscape.

56 H. C. Fanshawe, *The History of the Fanshawe Family* (Newcastle upon Tyne: A. Reid, 1927), 119.

3. Considering the Starter Collection: Fanshawe, Family, and Imported Knowledge

Abstract: While scholars have addressed the impact of diplomatic travels on Ann Fanshawe's recipe collection, this chapter concentrates on the cosmopolitan nature of the recipes Fanshawe inherited from her mother, Margaret Harrison. As the wife of John Harrison, a customs farmer who oversaw activities at the London docks, Margaret Harrison had access to many imported ingredients, which found their way into Fanshawe's 1651 starter recipe manuscript. Comparing recipes that Fanshawe attributes to "my mother" with those attributed to her husband's more rurally ensconced relatives, this chapters shows that the Harrison family's London experiences situate Fanshawe's starter collection in the world of trade and travel well before it ever left England.

Keywords: Wellcome MS7113; Margaret Harrison; John Harrison; recipe ingredients; international trade; imports

As Madeline Bassnett notes, early modern recipes recorded abroad capture English compilers in action as they engage with unfamiliar worlds. When recipes "contain foreign terminology, or otherwise make an effort to expose their provenance as being from elsewhere," Bassnett writes, "they actively demand that we receive and acknowledge the recipe as different; that, as readers, we engage with them textually as transcultural and transnational communications."[1] As Bassnett and many other scholars have shown, Ann

1 Madeline Bassnett, "A Language Not One's Own: Translational Exchange in Seventeenth-Century Englishwomen's Iberian Recipes," *Journal of Early Modern Cultural Studies* 19, no. 1 (2019): 2–3. Similarly, on the use of "newer" ingredients in recipes, see Sara Pennell, "Recipes and Reception: Tracking 'New World' Foodstuffs in Early Modern British Culinary Texts, c. 1650–1750," *Food & History* 7 (2009): 22–23, 32.

Nunn, Hillary M. *Recipes on the Move in Early Modern England and British North America: Domestic Medicine, Mobility, and Manuscript Culture*. Amsterdam: Amsterdam University Press, 2025.
DOI 10.5117/9789463723398_CH03

Fanshawe's recipe collection certainly makes this effort to reflect upon and incorporate her experiences living as an ambassador's wife in France, Portugal, and numerous other European locations. Amy L. Tigner and Melissa Schultheis, for example, examine ways that Fanshawe's recipes represent and modify cooking traditions and practices learned abroad;[2] David Goldstein, meanwhile, considers how Fanshawe's recipes contribute to our understanding of the era's notions of commensality.[3] These studies glean much of their insight from the recipes Fanshawe added to her manuscript during experiences in diplomatic missions in the 1660s. These fascinating entries, ranging from notes on perfuming gloves the Spanish way to her drawing of a chocolate pot, clearly show Fanshawe "engaging with a fluidly multicultural world and expressing an active and respectful curiosity" about its domestic habits.[4]

Much of Fanshawe's manuscript, however, reflects experiences with non-English cultures dating well before she undertook these well-documented diplomatic missions abroad. The recipes appearing in the earliest sections of her manuscript reflect engagement with a multicultural world, one revealing not just rural and cosmopolitan forces comingling but the gradual introduction of materials and mindsets gathered from international trade. Even the early recipes Fanshawe traces directly to members of her family show these influences. Alongside his note that entitles the book *Mrs. Fanshawes Booke of Receipts*, the scribe Joseph Averie dates the compilation's beginnings to December of 1651,[5] creating what Elaine Leong calls a "starter collection" in a "neat scribal hand, in contrast to the less practiced hands used to fill in the blank pages with additional recipes."[6] In Fanshawe's manuscript, Averie divides the book's pages into sections, with labels like "Physicks," "Cookery," and "How to

2 Amy L. Tigner, "Trans-Border Kitchens: Iberian Recipes in Seventeenth-Century English Manuscripts," *History of Retailing and Consumption* 5, no. 1 (2019): 51–70 and Melissa Schultheis, "A Culinary Embassy: Diplomatic Home Making in Lady Ann Fanshawe's *Booke of Receipts*," in *In the Kitchen, 1550–1800: Reading English Cooking at Home and Abroad*, eds. Madeline Bassnett and Hillary M. Nunn (Amsterdam: Amsterdam University Press, 2022), 197–217.

3 David B. Goldstein, *Eating and Ethics in Shakespeare: Staging Food and Drink in Early Modern England* (Cambridge: Cambridge University Press, 2013), 139–70.

4 Bassnett, "A Language Not One's Own," 4.

5 Ann Fanshawe, *Mrs. Fanshawes Booke of Receipts of Physickes Salues, Waters, Cordials, Preserves and Cookery*, 1678, Wellcome MS 7113, Wellcome Library, London, England, 3r. I have used the penciled-in folio numbers to cite pages in the Fanshawe recipe manuscript, because they are more consistently helpful even though they are smaller.

6 See Elaine Leong, *Recipes and Everyday Knowledge* (Chicago: University of Chicago Press, 2018), 21–22. For more on "starter collections," see Leong, *Recipes for Everyday Knowledge*, 21–23.

make Sirrups," and he begins the book's index.[7] Later additions largely followed Averie's divisions, though the index was only intermittently tended to. And indeed the compilation would grow. Not only did Fanshawe add to it during her travels; in 1678, she gave it to her daughter Katherine, who expanded it as well.

The well-earned scholarly focus on Fanshawe's later entries concentrates on their international flair, implying that the initial Averie-transcribed recipes embody a more homebound approach. Indeed, at first glance, the earliest entries in Fanshawe's recipe manuscript appear far more local in their concerns, and they may seem to be more geographically limited in their scope. Looking more carefully, however, these early recipes reflect the international character braided into Fanshawe's childhood experiences in London, as well as her own travels in the earliest years of her 1644 marriage. These Averie-recorded entries demonstrate a different sort of cultural engagement and curiosity, with their focus on family relationships allowing us heretofore unappreciated glimpses into the connections Ann Fanshawe's parents nourished not only with London's rich world of commerce, but international trade and colonial efforts as well.

The earliest recipes in Fanshawe's compilation reveal that the collection began with a diplomatic mission of its own: the integration of Fanshawe's own early experiences into the world of her husband's family. The Averie-inscribed pages of Fanshawe's recipe book seem at first glance to downplay her significant travels as a teenager and during the early days of her marriage. Instead, these pages work to anchor Fanshawe within her marital social network, incorporating recipes offered from relatives and friends, whose names appear as attributions in the margins, as a means to declare and solidify her connection within the Fanshawe family. Even though this collection's first pages are set down well after her marriage begins, those pre–1651 recipes illustrate the blending of Fanshawe's girlhood family with her husband's. The Averie-inscribed sections mingle the recipes Fanshawe inherited from her mother with those of her husband's relatives, often setting them side-by-side on the same page.

In fact, recipes from her husband's family dominate in these early manuscript sections, where they constitute the majority of recipe attributions; her collection thus complicates the oft-repeated notion that starter collections emphasize recipes passed from mothers to daughters.[8] In sheer numbers,

7 Fanshawe, *Mrs. Fanshawes Booke of Receipts*, 1678, Wellcome MS 7113, 4r, 126r, 174r.

8 For discussion of recipe manuscripts as a preoccupation for entire families, rather than women only, see Leong, *Recipes and Everyday Knowledge*, 23–31, and Wendy Wall, *Recipes*

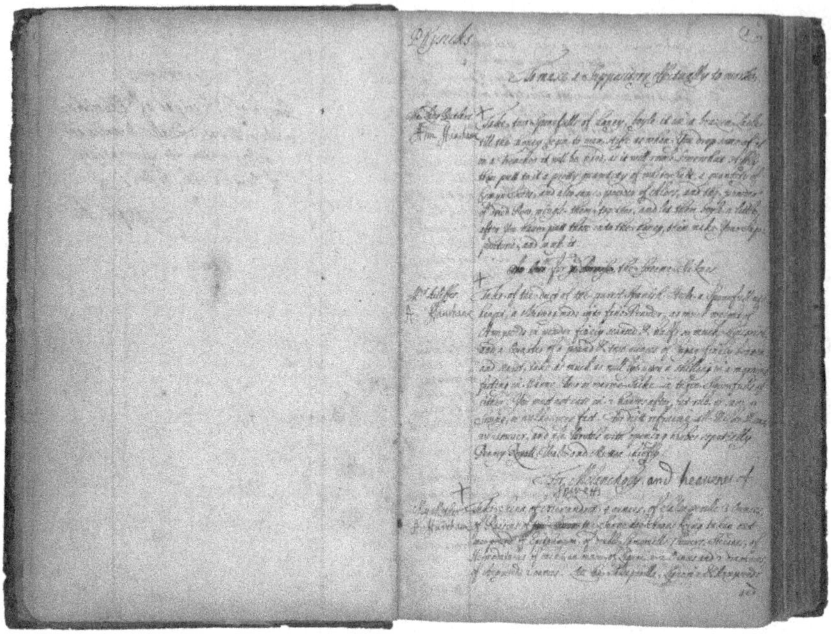

Figure 3. The first page of *Mrs. Fanshawes Book of Receipts*, 1678, Wellcome MS 7113. Courtesy of the Wellcome Collection.

recipes attributed to Ann's mother dominate in the first sections, but the book does not begin with them; instead, the first recipe is credited to her sister-in-law, Lady Joan Butler, and the second is from a Mrs. Ailiffes (likely Ayloffe), while the third is from "My Mother" (figure 3).[9] Counting the attributions recorded in the Averie sections as a whole, moreover, we can see that there are more pointing to her in-laws as sources than to her own mother.[10] This blending of her in-laws' practices into her own inherited cooking traditions constitutes a kind of diplomacy of its own, allowing us to see how Fanshawe carefully weaves her present and past together in a recipe book that bolsters her connections to members of her husband's family.

for Thought: Knowledge and Taste in the Early Modern Kitchen (Philadelphia: University of Pennsylvania Press, 2015), 191–93.

9 Fanshawe, *Mrs. Fanshawes Booke of Receipts*, 1678, Wellcome MS 7133, 4r. For useful genealogical trees featuring intermarriage between the Ayloffe and Fanshawe families before Ann's birth, see H. C. Fanshawe, *The History of the Fanshawe Family* (Newcastle upon Tyne: A. Reid, 1927).

10 Of the recipes in Averie's hand, Fanshawe attributes forty to her mother and fifty to her in-laws. Such numerical analyses were mentioned in an unpublished conference paper by Hillary Nunn and Melissa Schultheis, "Using the Methods of Our Manuscripts" (Conference Paper, *Modern Language Association Conference*, New York, NY, January 2018).

In early 1653, soon after the date Averie records as the start of his transcription, Fanshawe moved from London with her husband and young family to Tankersley Park, a Yorkshire house not twenty miles from where Ann's mother Margaret was born in Derbyshire.[11] Though Ann had married Richard Fanshawe in 1644, at no previous point in her marriage had she been able to settle comfortably into a home of her own, and the family's arrival in Yorkshire finally permitted her the chance to establish her own household. The setting contrasted markedly with Fanshawe's previous homes—she had grown up in London but, as a teenager, fled hurriedly with her sister and Royalist father to Oxford; after her marriage, she had lived in France, Ireland, and Spain, not to mention the months she spent living with sympathetic families in London and on England's southwest coast and Channel Islands.[12] These experiences, just like her later diplomatic travels of the 1660s, influenced her recipe compilation, though in a far subtler way.

Along with the documentation of travels apparent in her recipe book—entitled *Mrs. Fanshawes Booke of Receipts of Physickes Salues, Waters, Cordials, Preserves and Cookery* on its opening pages—Fanshawe also wrote a formal memoir in manuscript, presented in 1676 to her son Richard. Begun more than two decades after she began her recipe compilation, *The Memoirs of Ann, Lady Fanshawe* looks back on her life, including passages describing her efforts to establish some security for her growing family after the chaos of the Civil War. Though she aims to describe for her son "the most remarkable actions and accidents of your family, as well as those of more eminent ones of your father and my life," she devotes the majority of the *Memoir*'s opening to her husband's, rather than to her own, family's genealogy.[13] Ann's implication to her son that the Fanshawes are "your family," Katherine Hodgkin

11 Loftis provides a useful chronology of the events of Fanshawe's life, including the many places she resided with her family. Fanshawe had arrived in London from Ireland in 1651, the same year Averie began writing out her recipe manuscript. See Anne Fanshawe, *The Memoirs of Ann, Lady Fanshawe*, in *The Memoirs of Anne, Lady Halkett and Ann, Lady Fanshawe*, ed. John Loftis (Oxford: Clarendon, 1979), 95–99.

12 Fanshawe's life is unusually well documented, and her life writing has resulted in a wide variety of scholarly work. An entry is devoted to her in the *Oxford Dictionary of National Biography*—see Peter Davidson, "Fanshawe [*née* Harrison], Ann, Lady Fanshawe," in *Oxford Dictionary of National Biography* (Oxford: Oxford University Press, 2004)—and she is the subject of a popular biography; see Lucy Moore, *Lady Fanshawe's Receipt Book: The Life and Times of a Civil War Heroine* (London: Atlantic, 2017). Her family has long been the subject of much scholarly attention as well. See H. C. Fanshawe, *The History of the Fanshawe Family.*

13 Unless otherwise noted, all references to Fanshawe's memoirs are to Ann Fanshawe, *The Memoirs of Ann, Lady Fanshawe*, in *The Memoirs of Anne, Lady Halkett and Ann, Lady Fanshawe*, ed. John Loftis (Oxford: Clarendon, 1979), 101–92. This reference is Fanshawe, *The Memoirs of Ann, Lady Fanshawe*, 101.

argues, suggests that "however completely [Fanshawe] has identified her interests with those of her marriage family, she is not one of them."[14] Such a declaration reinforces Ann's perception of a need for her recipe book to bridge gaps between her natal family and her husband's.

The *Memoir* provides a natural complement to the recipe manuscript, offering a more conventional narrative, even if brief, of Fanshawe's early life and marriage. Born Ann Harrison on March 25, 1625, Fanshawe took charge of her father's household at the age of fifteen, after the death of her mother. Soon after, her father was imprisoned, leaving the once well-off family struggling financially. She married Richard Fanshawe, her second cousin, in 1644, and later declared that "what ever was reall happiness, God gave it me in him."[15] Unlike many Royalist wives, Fanshawe traveled with her husband as he fled parliamentary forces, following him to Ireland, Paris, and Spain before returning with him to London in 1651, where he was briefly imprisoned.[16] Only then, after seven years of marriage, did Fanshawe take advantage of the pause in her travels to start work on her recipe book—something that many brides would have done far earlier in their marriages, if not even before moving from their childhood homes; once the family moved to Yorkshire in early 1653, she finally had the chance to put those recipes to work in a household of her own.

Looking Abroad, Forging a Domestic Identity

The recipe book's mission of solidifying family identity, entwining the Fanshawe and the Harrison sides, is facilitated by Fanshawe's experiences forging connections between her own culture and the faraway places she had so recently lived. The collection's Averie sections comfortably blend local and imported ingredients, and this eases the juxtaposition of Harrison family recipes with those from the less cosmopolitan Fanshawe network her husband grew up in. The result is the creation of a common ground

14 Katherine Hodgkin, "Women, Memory and Family History in Seventeenth-Century England," in *Memory before Modernity: Practices of Memory in Early Modern Europe*, eds., Erika Kuijpers, Judith Pollman, Johannes Müller, and Jasper van der Steen (Leiden: Brill, 2013), 306.

15 Fanshawe, *The Memoirs of Ann, Lady Fanshawe*, edited by Loftis, 103. The fact that Ann and Richard were second cousins means their genealogies overlapped several generations earlier. Ann's connection to the Fanshawes comes through her mother's line, and those relatives appear to have been less a part of her childhood.

16 See Loftis's chronology for specifics, in Fanshawe, *The Memoirs of Ann, Lady Fanshawe*, edited by Loftis, 95–99.

for their extended families in a single household manuscript. The Averie sections of the manuscript carry traces of its owner's early time abroad, and these elements establish the collection's welcoming air. Commenting on Fanshawe's enduring links to the people she meets abroad, Anne Holloway and Ramona Wray identify Fanshawe's intense, immediate connection with Ireland and Spain in 1649–50 as a family feeling, "a sense of national-cultural consanguinity"[17] that resulted in lasting attachments. Such attachments, in their view, make Fanshawe's early travels in Spain a motivating force for starting her recipe book, demonstrating "cultural assimilation and imaginative engagement" while "highlight[ing] the emancipatory effects of geographical displacement."[18] Travel, in other words, loosens the local bonds that might have otherwise dictated Fanshawe's lived domestic practice.

Fanshawe, moreover, never leaves these overseas attachments completely behind; on the contrary, her recipes suggest a bodily, sensory pull to locations abroad even after her return to England. While medical theories would assume Fanshawe would thrive best when back in the humorally familiar lands of her birth, Fanshawe nonetheless remembers, and seeks to recreate, the sensory experiences associated with her time spent outside of England. She sometimes links the recipes acquired during these experiences with her fellow Royalists abroad, thus lending them an English air despite their roots in exile. Her insertion of recipes from her English compatriots in France, Sir Kenelm Digby and Susan Feilding, Lady Denbigh[19]—as well her

17 Anne Holloway and Ramona Wray, "'O daughter ... forget your people and your father's house': Early Modern Women Writers and the Spanish Imaginary," *Bulletin of Spanish Studies* 9 (2016): 1396.

18 Holloway and Wray, "'O daughter ... forget your people and your father's house,'" 1403.

19 Her compilation contains, by Archer's count, fifteen recipes linked to Susan Feilding, Lady Denbigh, with whom Fanshawe served at Queen Henrietta Maria's court in France in 1648. While these fifteen recipes make Lady Denbigh "the most significant source outside of Ann's immediate family," her contributions do not appear in the sections Averie produced, though the recipes may well have been in Fanshawe's possession at the time those recipes were transcribed. On the other hand, of the eight recipes associated with Sir Kenelm Digby, seven appear in Averie's handwriting. Archer points out that Digby's 1669 *The Closet of Sir Kenelm Digby Opened* contains "My Lady *Fanshaws* way of feeding Capons, Pullets, Hens, Chickens or Turkies," which does not appear in Fanshawe's own collection. See Jayne Elisabeth Archer, "'An Offering to her Memory': Healing, Motherhood, and Identity in the Manuscript Remains of Lady Ann Fanshawe," in *Identities in Early Modern English Writing: Religion, Gender, Nation*, ed. Lorna Fitzsimmons (Turnhout: Brepols, 2014), 6:134. Perhaps it is this omission that leads the editor of the 1907 printing of the *Memoir* to conclude the recipe "belongs no doubt to Lady Elizabeth Fanshawe, of Ware Park, and not to the wife of Sir Richard, to whom it has been ascribed." See Ann Fanshawe, *The Memoirs of Ann, Lady Fanshawe, Wife of Sir Richard Fanshawe, bart., 1600–72*, ed. Herbert Charles Fanshawe (London: J. Lane, 1907), 288. Other unrelated family friends are

incorporation of recipes from her 1650 trip to Madrid in a later section of Spanish recipes sewn into the manuscript—marries the foods, perfumes, and medicines encountered during her travels with those already rooted in her English family and environment.[20]

While Fanshawe's stay in Yorkshire after her marriage's initial rootlessness is brief, it marks the start of her recipe collection's formalization, as well as a convenient stopping point from which to consider the impact of her early life and travels on her healthcare practices. Indeed, travel and trade constituted a key factor in Fanshawe's pre–1651 life, even though she seemed firmly rooted in London. Her family's commercial connections shaped her sense of home healthcare, even though her experience of places abroad was not firsthand. Living in London, the daughter of a man who earned his notable wealth working as a customs farmer and therefore depending on foreign trade, Fanshawe was steeped in conversations about travel and the imports it generated. Her London origins permeate the book's earlier recipes, which often carry labels attributing them to Fanshawe's mother Margaret. Recipes for the medical treatments linked to Margaret bear the marks of London's status as an international trading hub, combining native plants with imported ingredients to concoct a wide range of cures.

With these detailed instructions for amalgamating imported and local ingredients, the earliest entries in Fanshawe's recipe book prefigure what Stacy Alaimo and others have dubbed "material memoirs," which treat experience as "data" that allow personal experiences to be interpreted "through a scientific lens." Alaimo writes that "these trans-corporeal autobiographies insist that the self is constituted by material agencies that are simultaneously biological, political, and economic."[21] Detailing how personal,

named in the Averie section as well. Lady Browne, wife of the English ambassador in Paris Sir Richard Browne, offers two culinary recipes (Fanshawe, *Mrs. Fanshawe's Booke of Receipts*, 1678, Wellcome MS 7113, 134v, 135v). Browne, related to Fanshawe by marriage, was father-in-law to John Evelyn, who also recorded some of Ann Fanshawe's recipes in his collection. See Geoffrey Smith, "Surviving the Cavalier Winter: The Experience of Richard and Ann Fanshawe," *Parergon* 32, no. 3 (2015), 109–10 and Goldstein, *Eating and Ethics*, 139–70.

20 Curiously, Fanshawe makes no obvious mention of Irish sources, perhaps because of the physical discomfort she endured there. During the escape from Cork, Fogarty writes, "Fanshawe's throbbing, broken wrist and pregnant body encrypt her feelings of vulnerability and fear that otherwise are censored and unexpressed." See Ann Fogarty, "Reading Dislocation and Emotion in the Writings of Alice Thornton, Ann Fanshawe, and Barbara Blaugdone," in *Women's Life Writing and Early Modern Ireland*, eds. Julie A. Eckerle and Naomi McAreavey (Lincoln: University of Nebraska Press, 2019), 66.

21 Stacy Alaimo, *Bodily Natures: Science, Environment, and the Material Self* (Bloomington and Indianapolis: University of Indiana Press, 2010), 87.

bodily histories and the story of the environment overlap, Alaimo points to Susanne Antonetta's blend of ecological research and personal narrative in her memoir *Body Toxic*. "Autobiography," Alaimo writes, "becomes profoundly biological as bodies and selves are constructed from the very stuff of the toxic places they have inhabited."[22] In Fanshawe's work, toxic elements at first appear primarily social and political in nature, as she flees England and then Ireland in search of refuge from parliamentary troops, but her recipes carry with them traces of the bodily changes—often positive—that result from her journeys to different countries. These changes run deeper than the externally visual markers of pregnancy and even male dress that she describes in recounting her travels.[23] Rather, the materials she ingests while outside of her English homeland change into her body as she encounters them. The medicines, foods, and environments of these places, in Alaimo's words "take up residence within the body"—in early modern terms, permeating Fanshawe's ever-changing humoral constitution—and in the process "the supposedly inert 'background' of place becomes the active substance of self."[24] And it is Fanshawe's recipe manuscript, not her memoir, that reveals how these travels seep into her body through the medical practices she adopts abroad and preserves for later household use.

The Harrisons, at Home and Abroad

Despite the years Fanshawe spent abroad before formally beginning her collection, many scholars read Fanshawe's recipe manuscript as starting with her mother, Margaret Harrison, who died much earlier, when her daughter was a teenager. This emphasis underscores in many studies the matrilineal narrative often associated with recipe exchanges. Sara Pennell writes that recipe books traveled "along female kin lines" and served as "inter-generational routes for female-to-female communication"; her work, however, is careful to show the influence men had on compiling these books.[25] More recently, Wendy Wall has pointed out that Ann Fanshawe, in

22 Alaimo, *Bodily Natures*, 102.

23 On Fanshawe's cross-dressing during a sea voyage, see Mary Beth Rose, *Gender and Heroism in Early Modern English Literature* (Chicago: University of Chicago Pres, 2002), 68–70 and Holloway and Wray, "'O daughter ... forget your people and your father's house,'" 1397–98.

24 Alaimo, *Bodily Natures*, 102.

25 Sara Pennell, "Perfecting Practice?: Women Manuscript Recipes and Knowledge in Early Modern England," in *Early Modern Women's Manuscript Writing: Selected Papers from the Trinity/ Trent Colloquium*, eds. Victoria E. Burke and Jonathan Gibson (Basingstoke: Ashgate, 2004), 240.

passing her recipes down to her daughter Katherine, enabled her daughter "to imagine three generations of women's practices in the family, including those undertaken by Katherine's sister ... mother, and grandmother Margaret."[26] While we know that Fanshawe's book remained within the female line, it is clear that men take their place in this system of recipe manuscript inheritance as well. Elaine Leong points out that sons as well as daughters were named as owners of these books, and entries in these recipe collections reflect domestic knowledge from men as well as women. As a result, Leong argues, these collections are family books as much as they are women's legacies. At the same time, Leong too suggests that Fanshawe's book began as a copy of her mother Margaret Harrison's collection.[27]

As Lucy Moore sees it, Harrison's early death made her recipes key to Fanshawe's recollections of the idyllic days of her childhood. Moore imagines the teenage Ann, fleeing her prosperous home in London to Oxford to avoid parliamentarian violence, as grabbing:

> only what she could carry on horseback: some clothes, quilted or fur-lined against the cold, and a sheaf of her mother's receipts that she had copied out as a childhood handwriting exercise, thrust into a cloak bag. Today, refugees carry their world in their mobile phones—contacts, memories, plans and dreams. For Ann, the world she hoped to remember and recreate was in that slim bundle of papers.[28]

Though there is little evidence to support the details of Moore's scene, the nostalgia she pinpoints echoes many accounts of recipes acting as attachments to family line. This image of the young Ann struggling to retain a sense of home, safely anchored in English traditions, however, overlooks the substantial international flavor of Fanshawe's early life. The daughter of Sir John Harrison and Margaret Fanshawe Harrison, Fanshawe claims to "have little knowledge" of her father's family, but she knew that he came to London from Lancashire to serve Sir John Wolstenholme, who "gave him a small place in the Custome House."[29] Ann's mother Margaret, meanwhile, was sent from her home at Fanshawe's Gate in Derbyshire to London, where she worked in Wolstenholme's household until she married Harrison, in 1616.[30]

26 Wall, *Recipes for Thought*, 191.
27 Leong, *Recipes and Everyday Knowledge*, 23.
28 Moore, *Lady Fanshawe's Receipt Book*, 1–2.
29 Fanshawe, *The Memoirs of Ann, Lady Fanshawe*, edited by Loftis, 110.
30 H. C. Fanshawe, *The History of the Fanshawe Family*, 42.

Harrison's abilities and connections soon led to his success as a customs farmer—that is, a businessman licensed by the crown to collect customs duties from those importing and exporting goods from the port of London.[31] Ann thus grew up in a London household that depended on international trade for its livelihood, since her father worked in his position for over twenty years, starting in 1620 (five years before Ann's birth). Harrison's work with importers even drew him to invest in overseas ventures such as the Virginia Company and the East India Company, suggesting an even greater engagement with international commerce.[32]

These connections meant that the Harrison household was steeped in a world of imports and finance, even when its members were firmly rooted in England. Harrison's work provided the family with an ample income and a huge library, stocked with lawbooks and at least two well-worn medical texts, including a copy of Gerard's *Herball*.[33] Margaret ministered to the health of her household, calling not just on these texts but on the materials that her husband's position allowed her. Fanshawe describes her mother not only as a great beauty, but as a charitable woman who "drest many wounds of miserable people when she had health, and when that fall'd, as it did often, she caused her servant to supply that place."[34]

The Harrisons' commercial connections were not their only links to the era's globalizing forces, thanks to the distinct but largely undiscerned presence of Ann's uncle, Jamestown colonist George Harrison, brother of Sir John Harrison. The allure of the Americas—the material wealth to be earned there, as well as the adventures and dangers it represented—also shades the family's concerns, and eventually Fanshawe's 1651 recipes. While George Harrison spent a relatively short time in Virginia, arriving in 1622 and dying there two years later, he maintained correspondence during that time with Ann's father. Born in 1625, Ann could never have met her uncle, yet his impact lingered through the family's business well beyond his

31 Robert Ashton, "Revenue Farming under the Early Stuarts," *Economic History Review* 8, no. 3 (1956), 310.

32 Mary Freer Keeler, *The Long Parliament, 1640–1641: A Biographical Study of Its Members* (Philadelphia: American Philosophical Society, 1954), 205 and Simon Healy, "HARRISON, John (c.1589–1669), of St. Olave's, Hart Street, London; later of Balls Park, Herts. and Beaumont, Lancs," in *The Parliament: The House of Commons 1604–1629*, eds. Andrew Thrush and John P. Ferris (Cambridge: Cambridge University Press, 2010).

33 F. J. Levy, "How Information Spread among the Gentry, 1550–1640," *Journal of British Studies* 21, no. 2 (1982): 29–31. The law books also suggest Harrison's efforts at attempting to reform the system that led to unstable relationships between the Crown and customs farmers. See Ashton, "Revenue Farming under the Early Stuarts," 310–22.

34 Fanshawe, *The Memoirs of Ann, Lady Fanshawe*, edited by Loftis, 109.

death. When George died as the result of a duel, he left his brother to tend to his Virginia land claims. Given that her father John Harrison was also an investor in the Virginia Company, it follows that a lasting connection would have existed between family matters and business of the Jamestown colony.

The young colonist George even sought to involve Fanshawe's mother in American commerce, suggesting in a letter dated January 24, 1623, that Margaret Harrison "should make a good private adventure" by sending along wines, butter, cheese, and soap to Virginia, presumably at least partially for resale, by the next ship out. Even though the letter's news is otherwise grim, with reports of a massacre and sickness hinting that "God has cast a heavy hand upon them," George managed to send three hogsheads of tobacco back to England.[35] Later that year, on September 16, 1623, a shipment with George's name on it landed in Virginia, containing the requested cheese and much more, including sugar and spices from other colonies. The paperwork attached to this gift from the London Harrisons makes clear that the cheese, as well as oil and aquavitae, were purchased rather than homemade.[36] While the document has John Harrison's name on it, rather than Margaret's, she could have played a role in procuring the goods, in accordance with George's earlier suggestion. As Alexander Brown tells it, though, this shipment of potentially lifesaving supplies ironically brought about George Harrison's early death; it led to his lethal duel with the merchant Richard Stephens, who delivered Harrison "a cut in the leg which did somewhat grieve him and 14 days after he departed this life." Curiously, Stephens was not held responsible because the "Doctor and Chirgions did open [Harrison's] bodie upon the Juries request and they found it very fowle" and ruled "he could not have lived long."[37] Apparently, whatever killed him—presumably a rottenness acquired during his time in Virginia—had already taken up residence in his body, hastening his premature demise far away from his place of birth.

While George Harrison's death in 1624 meant that he never met his niece, his life epitomized the colonial impulses permeating Ann Fanshawe's surroundings in her parents' home in St. Olave's parish in London. The settling of George's will lingered, with Ann's father overseeing the disposal of his brother's rather substantial property in Virginia through a power of attorney, so it is quite possible that conversations about life and land in Virginia seeped

35 "America and West Indies: January 1623," in *Calendar of State Papers, Colonial, America and West Indies*, 1:35–37.

36 Susan Myra Kingsbury, ed., *The Records of the Virginia Company* (Washington, DC, 1906–35), 4:278–81.

37 Alexander Brown, *The First Republic in America* (Boston: Hughton, 1898), 582.

into Ann's early childhood world.[38] Family friends and distant relations cited in the Averie recipes had similar tales to tell about relatives in the American colonies; for example, two members of the Newce family were instrumental in settlements that became Newport News in Virginia, and a Mrs. Newce provides two recipes in Fanshawe's collection.[39] Talk of far-off Virginia, moreover, mixed with the language of the custom house and the materials that made their way into the family's surroundings. As George's request for goods makes clear, the Harrisons had access to large quantities of both domestic and imported materials, and the recipes that Ann later attributes to "my Mother" in her book reflect those cosmopolitan roots. And that access, along with the goods and stories brought home on a daily basis from John Harrison's business, helped to give rise to a heavy reliance on imported ingredients in the recipes of Fanshawe's youth, acquired long before she ever left England.

Native Soils: Importation and the Origins of Medical Ingredients

Even though the first home that Fanshawe's 1651 starter collection would have known was in England, it already reflected the influences of her time in Ireland and Spain, as well as her mother's London access to goods from around the world, her father's work with imports and importers, and the dealings surrounding his brother George's life and death in Virginia. This extensive geographical and social reach leaves traces of the family's international experience on the compilation well before Fanshawe undertook much of her life abroad as wife of a diplomat. These starter recipes, and the family's temporary Tankersley Park location, have earned little attention from scholars of her recipe books who might see it as conflicting with the rather adventurous, even

38 Francis Burton Harrison offers a concise history of George Harrison's life in the historical record, usefully extending the discussion to John and his family. At times, however, he confuses these Harrisons with another family of Harrisons, whose Virginia line gave rise to William Henry Harrison, the ninth president of the United States. See Francis Burton Harrison, "Harrisons in Virginia during the Reign of James I (Concluded)," *The Virginia Magazine of History and Biography* 51, no. 4 (1943): 326–38.

39 Mrs. Newce offers "An approued medecine for the convulsion fitts" and "A Diett Drink." See Fanshawe, *Mrs. Fanshawes Booke of Receipts*, 1678, Wellcome MS 7113, 6v–7r. Mrs. Newce may have been born Mary Fanshawe; Mary's son Thomas Newse was appointed to the Virginia council and died in Virginia in 1623. George Sandys, meanwhile, identified Sir William Newse, brother of Thomas, as founder of Newport News in 1621; William returned to England. See Lyon Gardiner Tyler, *Encyclopedia of Virginia Biography* (New York: Lewis Historical Publishing, 1915), 1:85–86, 91.

swashbuckling image Fanshawe otherwise enjoys. In some ways, she seems to have deemphasized this time in her life as well; as we shall see, Fanshawe's years sequestered with her children in the countryside occupy far less space in the memoir than her stories of political intrigue on the Continent.

That said, the medical recipes traced to her mother in these initial sections of the manuscript are far from basic, often in contrast to the cures attributed to members of her husband's family. At times, the sophistication comes through in the framing of these recipes, as in Margaret Harrison's instructions for "The King of France his Balsome." Despite a title that implies access to the cures of international royalty, the concoction itself resembles the green ointment recipes Lady Grace Castleton and her Yorkshire neighbors describe. Harrison's recipe, in Averie's hand, reads as follows:

> Take Red Sage, and Rue each one pound, of young Bay Leaves and Wormwood of each ½ a pound, doe not wash them, but picke, wipe and cut them very small, and beate them well in a Stone Morter, take 3 pound of Sheepes Suett hot from the Sheepe, mince it small & breake it with those herbes till it be all of one coulour; then putt all into a faire boule with a pottle of the best oile Olive, worke all together till it become alike, then putt it into an Earthen pott well stopt with Parchment and waxe for 8 dayes. Then seethe all in a panne with a soft Fire. When it is sodden putt to it 4 ounces of the oile of Spike. Then straine, it thorow a Canvas Strainer into a pott, couer it with parchment, and with a Leather upon that; In the boyling of it take heed that it burne not, for the avoyding whereof putt 2 or 3 drops still in a Sawcer, and when it is greene as the Emrod it is enough
>
> This is excellent for all Aches, or paines of the Head that come of Cold black wooll being dipt in it, and stopping the Eares, for shrinking of Sinewes, or Ague Cakes being chaft in against The Fire, & a Cloth dipt hott in the same applied to the Place.[40]

The recipe, like many with Yorkshire roots described in chapter 2, assumes that the maker can access "Suett hot form the Sheepe" as well as black wool. These descriptions bring a Northern tinge to the recipe, suggesting a preparation that could recall Margaret Harrison's rural childhood at Fanshawe Gate despite its title's invocation of the King of France. The title, however, is not the only hint of a more cosmopolitan outlook. The resulting

40 Fanshawe, *Mrs. Fanshawes Booke of Receipts*, 1678, Wellcome MS 7113, 30r.

ointment has the same color as other green ointments, but its green is phrased in less pastoral terms—it is "greene as the Emrod," or emerald, resembling an imported jewel rather than the products of the field. The recipe thus presumes its maker occupies a place where sheep butchering and rare gems—or at least the knowledge of them—coexist.

Margaret Harrison's thirty-six medicinal recipes reflect a greater variety of ingredients and methods than those Ann Fanshawe attributes to her sisters-in-law. Alice Fanshawe Bedells, Richard Fanshawe's sister, who is associated with over a dozen medical recipes in Averie's 1651 section, contributes concise recipes that often rely on local animals; her "An Oyntment for Burning with Gunpowder or Scalding with Water" contains four ingredients—boar's grease, leeks, sheep dung, and goose dung—while her "For a stroke or Bruise in the Eye" uses only one: a live pigeon, whose "great Veine of the | Wing" should be pierced in such a way that "the Blood Spring out of the Veine."[41] On the other hand, the eight medical recipes from Joan Fanshawe Boteler—the manuscript's "Lady Butler," another of Richard Fanshawe's sisters—incorporate a great number of imports, but suggest caution in doing so. Her recipes for a drink "to be taken in the Spring to purge the Blood," for example, calls for rhubarb, oranges, cloves, and raisins; she even offers a distilled "Spirett of Amber Gris."[42] At the same time, though, she relies heavily on locally produced ingredients like honey in her recipes. Lady Butler, it appears, was willing to incorporate imports into the medicines produced in her kitchen, but she generally tempered them with ingredients from lands she knew firsthand.

With their blending of local and imported ingredients, the medical recipes Averie records in Ann Fanshawe's book reflect a willingness to modify of the Hippocratic principles of humoral healthcare. The insistence that bodies thrive best when treated with ingredients produced in the place of their birth—a notion fundamental to guidelines set out in the still-influential treatise *Airs, Waters, Places*—undergoes perpetual challenge in Fanshawe's recipe manuscript, even in its early pages. As we shall see, she collects recipes whose ingredients, and cited contributors, honor the Fanshawe's rural roots, but those cures exist alongside instructions for creating medicines that rely upon imported raw materials. Those imported ingredients, moreover, often blend with homegrown botanicals. The afflictions these recipes treat also reflect local patterns of illness, rather than ailments acquired as a result of travel. Fanshawe's manuscript, in short,

41 Fanshawe, *Mrs. Fanshawes Booke of Receipts*, 1678, Wellcome MS 7113, 32v.

42 Fanshawe, *Mrs. Fanshawes Booke of Receipts*, 1678, Wellcome MS 7113, 5v, 81r.

shows a willingness to make room for new cures, even when those cures challenge long-held convictions regarding the entanglements between humans to their natural surroundings.

The medical recipes that Fanshawe labels as her mother's take access to imports as a given, incorporating anise, carraway, nutmeg, and ginger without highlighting their foreign origins. In fact, Margaret Harrison's medical recipes—those, that is, attributed to "My Mother" and appearing in Averie's hand in Fanshawe's manuscript—commonly presume the availability of fresh botanical ingredients while also calling for knowledge of specific imported herbs and materials. Sometimes, the preparations call exclusively for imports. For example, the very first recipe labeled as coming from "My Mother"—a preparation for "For Melancholy and heavenes of spiritts"—begins with the requirement of "Sena of Alexandria 4 ounces, of Salsaperilla 3 Ounces, | of Raisins of the Sunne the Stones being taken out | one pound."[43] Such a blend of imported ingredients reflects not just an increasing volume of trade but suggests the affordability of even the most hard-to-find of materials.

The imported materials Margaret Harrison's recipes call for are commonly listed in the "Drugs" and "Groceries" categories of the royally approved taxation tables her husband would have consulted in his own work at the London Customs House. The names of many imports, then, would have been common vocabulary for Fanshawe's parents, and perhaps for the wider household as well. While the taxation tables were regularly updated before the Interregnum, the 1642 *Rates of Marchandizes* provided the most current tables at the time Averie began his work on the recipe manuscript in 1651.[44] Filling eight pages with taxation rates for ingredients ranging from acacia to zedoary, or white turmeric, the "Drugs" tables in the 1642 booklet specify levies on imports ranging from "Ambergreece black or gray the ounce," "Scorpions the piece," and "Mechoacan the pound" (a Mexican morning glory used as a purgative); the smaller "Grocery" category, meanwhile, details the taxes on spices such as cinnamon, mace, and dried fruits, while devoting most of a page to different sorts of sugar reaching the ports.[45]

43 Fanshawe, *Mrs. Fanshawes Booke of Receipts*, 1678, Wellcome MS 7113, 4r; "and heaveness of spirits" is in a separate hand, perhaps added by Fanshawe or her daughter Katherine.

44 *The Rates of Merchandizes. That is to Say, the Subsidy of Tonnage, the Subsidy of Poundage, and the Subsidy of Woollen, Cloths, or Old Drapery* (London, 1642). A 1635 version of the tables would have been the version in play at the time of Margaret Harrison's death in 1640. See *The Rates of Marchandizes as they are Set Downe in the Book of Rates* (London, 1635).

45 *The Rates of Merchandizes* (1642), 14–22 and 31–32.

While both the senna and sarsaparilla of Margaret Harrison's recipe for melancholy are listed in *The Rates of Merchandize*, its tables reflect little knowledge of the different varieties available, listing only "Sarsaparilla the pound" and "Sena the pound."[46] The two plants were among the most commonly imported drugs in the sixteenth and seventeenth centuries, though, as Patrick Wallis points out, those handling the trade may not have been attuned to variations in the quality—something perhaps not unexpected when volumes of imports were rising steadily.[47] The recipe calls for "Sena of Alexandria"—the most prized variety, according to Gerard, who declares "the best is brought from Alexandria and Egypt." In fact, he is quick to note that the plant "hardly groweth in high and low Germany, neither in England: it prospereth in hot Regions, and cannot away with cold."[48] Similarly, Gerard stresses that, even if sarsaparilla can be grown in Europe, its survival and effectiveness depend on the soil in which it grows.

While the rate book offers no sense of the differences that come with the origins of sarsaparilla, Gerard is clear that plants with the greatest effectiveness thrive in the Americas; his sense of where in America, however, is less clear. He declares that "Zarza Parilla, or the prickly Binde weed of America, groweth in Peru a prouince of America, in Virginia, and in diuers other places both in the East and West Indies."[49] Though George Harrison never mentions sending any sarsaparilla from Virginia to his London relatives, it was among the goods imported from Jamestown in the colony's earliest days.[50] Gerard's account, taken alongside knowledge of the Virginia colony, allows English consumers to imagine themselves using a medicinal plant approved, if not harvested, by their countrymen. This is especially true when Gerard connects the plant to John White, the artist whose watercolors were reprinted in Hariot's *Brief History of Virginia*, a text that offered the first glimpse of America to many readers:

46 *The Rates of Merchandizes* (1642), 21.

47 Wallis shows that both sarsaparilla and senna routinely ranked among the ten most valuable imported drug substances at London ports. Patrick Wallis, "Exotic Drugs and English Medicine: England's Drug Trade, c. 1550–c. 1800," *Social History of Medicine* 25, no. 1 (2012): 31.

48 John Gerard, *The Herball or Generall Historie of Plantes* (London, 1633), 1297.

49 Gerard, *The Herball or Generall Historie of Plantes*, 860.

50 Bruce notes, "In 1610, the Company in London, bearing in mind one of the principal objects for which the new settlement had been established, that is, to supply the people of England with many, if not all of the articles they were compelled at that time to import from abroad, instructed the authorities in Virginia to return to the mother country the following: sassafras root, bayberries, puccoon, galbrand, sarsaparilla, walnut oil, beaver, cod, oak and walnut trees, pines, pitch and tar, sturgeon, caviare and sounds for isinglass." See Philip Alexander Bruce, *Economic History of Virginia in the Seventeenth Century* (London: Macmillan, 1896), 261–62.

> White an excellent painter who carried very many people into Virginia (or after some Norembega) there to inhabit at which time hee did see thereof great plenty [of sarsaparilla], as he himselfe reported vnto me, with this bare description. It is (saith he) the root of a small shrubby tree, or hedge tree, such as are those of our country called Hawthorns hauing Leaues resembling those of Ivy, but the floures or fruit he remembreth not. It is moss certaine, that *Sarsaparilla* is the root of the Americane *Smilax aspera*, both by consent of most Writers, and by the relation of such as haue scene it growing there.[51]

Though growing in a faraway land, this sarsaparilla comes with an English stamp of approval. Yet Gerard's subsequent conversations confuse the plant's origins, connecting it most tightly to Peru. In his mind, the two American locations blend together, even as he remarks on how the place where a plant grows affects its potency. He proclaims:

> *Zarzaparilla* of Peru is a strange plant, and is brought vnto vs from the Countries of the new world called America; and such things as are brought from thence, although they also seeme and are like to those that grow in Europe, notwithstanding they doe often differ in vertue and operation: for the diuersitie of the soile and of the weather doth not only breed an alteration in the form, but doth most of all preuaile in making the vertues and qualities greater or lesser.[52]

As a result, when plants from hot places are moved to cool climates, they lose "force" and fragrance, and "Some things that are deadly and pernitious, being remoued wax milde, and are made wholesome." As a result, sarsaparilla from the Americas has "more force" because of "the temperature of the weather, and also through the nature of the soile."[53] Whether Harrison assumed a particular provider for her sarsaparilla, or whether Fanshawe minded such differences in her later preparation of her mother's recipe, we can never know; perhaps the women relied on their own skills to improvise with what was available.

The origins of local products matter as well, as we can see in Margaret Harrison's recipe "To make an Excellent opening and purging Drinke for the Liuer." Calling for imports like sarsaparilla, senna of Alexandria, and rhubarb,

51 Gerard, *The Herball or Generall History of Plantes*, 860.

52 Gerard, *The Herball or Generall History of Plantes*, 860–61.

53 Gerard, *The Herball or Generall History of Plantes*, 861.

the drink blends them with local herbs such as yellow dock, egrimony, and green scurvy grass.

> Take Salsaperilla, sliced and bruised, Polypodie of the Oake bruised Sena of Alexandria a little bruised, of each 4 ounces, Yellowe Docke rootes, washed, scraped bruised and the Pith taken forth of them, one ounce and a halfe, of Rhubard, halfe an ounce, thinne sliced of Nequo= quium, Egrimony and Maydenhaire, or each one handfull, Anniseeds Sweet fennel Seeds & Caraway seeds a little bruised of each one ounce. Liquorice scraped and bruised one ounce and a halfe, Mire all these to= gether, then take Greene Scruvy Grasse Leaues cleane pickt a pecke, Brooke Lime & Water Cresses of each halfe a Pecke ...[54]

One local ingredient—a mistletoe-like plant called polypody of oak—declares its best habitat in its name, which at least one unnamed apothecary takes seriously, according to his notes on the lectures delivered at the Worshipful Society of Apothecaries of London. He notes that, because polypody naturally "draws from the rotten mosse, & such thinges about the Oke | a fitting nourishment, & the like that hath & most commonly | in greater plenty in some old walls & ditch Banckes," students should source the plant from these locations. "I may advise you," he summarizes plainly, "gather the | hearbes where they grow naturally well likeing & strongest | in the tast & smell."[55] Plants raised in locations that allow them to thrive, he emphasizes, yield the most effective ingredients.

The recipe's rhubarb, on the other hand, is a mystery; the matter-of-fact notation of "Rhubarb, halfe an ounce" offers little help to a practitioner needing to decide which variety of this plant to use. A person with access to the well-stocked London apothecaries might assume the recipe required imported Chinese rhubarb, the variety with the murkiest origins but best reputation. Unlike an ingredient like polypody of oak, picked from trees growing in the practitioners' own environments, the roots of Chinese rhubarb plants often passed through a number of intermediary trading hubs in India, the Middle East, and the Mediterranean before arriving in England, suggesting that Europeans never saw Chinese rhubarb intact until the Jesuit Michal Boim offered the first description of the living plant in soil in the

54 Fanshawe, *Mrs. Fanshawes Booke of Receipts*, 1678, Wellcome MS 7113, 5r.

55 Worshipful Society of the Apothecaries of London, *Medical miscellany* [manuscript], ca. 1634, Folger MS E.a.5, Folger Shakespeare Library, Washington, DC, 97r.

1640s.[56] While rhubarb proves a vivid case regarding the partial knowledge of ingredients, it is by no means extraordinary, given the increasing use of imports; as Gerard muses, "It hath happened in this as in many other forreine medicines or simples, which though they be of great and frequent vse … yet haue we no certaine knowledge of the very place which produces them, nor of their exact manner of growing."[57]

By the time Fanshawe's first recipes were entered into her book, another, locally grown variety of rhubarb could have been available to her. The apothecary John Parkinson attempted to cultivate the plant from seeds sent to him from abroad by a "worthy Gentleman, Mr. Dr. Matth. Lister, one of the Kings Physitians." As Clifford M. Foust points out, Parkinson simultaneously labels the resulting rhubarb as identical to Chinese variety, remarking that it is "so like vnto the true Rubarbe, or the Rha of Pontus, both for forme and colour, that I dare say it is the very true Rubarbe," and as inferior to its imported counterpart. He blames the London environment for the plant's limited effectiveness, concluding that "our climate only mak[es] it lesse strong in working, lesse heauy, and lesse bitter in taste."[58] The plant may not have been effective, but the fact that it could be grown in kitchen gardens (and that Parkinson shared its seeds with members of the nobility) earned it a place in local practice. This variety, taken in conjunction with other local plants often called English Rhubarb,[59] meant that local practitioners could have chosen any one of a variety of rhubarbs to make their recipes. Depending on their locations and access, practitioners could have enjoyed several options to create a custom, fine-tuned recipe; others with fewer available choices, however, would have had to make do and hope for the best.

56 Clifford M. Foust, *Rhubarb: The Wondrous Drug* (Princeton: Princeton University Press, 1992), 23–24. Though by the early seventeenth century the East India Company's ships controlled cargoes for rhubarb from the time they left China to their arrival in London, the roots' travels within Asia to reach Chinese trading hubs after harvest remained obscure. Europeans looking for Chinese rhubarb "knew only of the lumps of spongy yet firm roots found in the marketplaces, those rather misshapen roots, black on the outside and reddish within, which were vulnerable to deterioration if not well dried." See Foust, *Rhubarb*, 17 as well as 5–6, and Wallis, "Exotic Drugs and English Medicine," 32.

57 Gerard, *The Herball or Generall History of Plantes*, 392.

58 John Parkinson, *Paradisi in Sole Paradisus Terrestris. or A Garden of All Sorts of Pleasant Flowers which our English Ayre will Permitt to be Noursed vp* (London, 1640), 484; quoted and modernized in Foust, *Rhubarb*, 19–20.

59 Bastard Rhubarb, or Monk's Rhubarb, are related native plants that also were available for use, and practitioners could easily have substituted them for imported rhubarb as well. The strength of the resulting medicines, of course, would vary wildly and require expertise in preparation. Gerard offers a discussion of the different plants labeled rhubarb; see Gerard, *The Herball or Generall History of Plantes*, 395–96.

Eating Dirt

The importance of the land that produces a recipe's ingredients comes into powerful focus in Lady Butler's "An excellent Medecine for any sore Mouth or Throat." The recipe, linked to Ann Fanshawe's sister-in-law, appears in Averie's hand in the Fanshawe manuscript's opening "Physicks" section. Like other recipes associated with Lady Butler, this one at first glance seems to combine an easily available, domestically sourced ingredient—honey—with an imported one. But this seemingly simple recipe betrays a hidden mystery about the ingredients' places of origin:

> Take as much Bole Armeniack as the weight of a groat,
> mingle it with ½ a Spoonfull of honey. Let the Patient
> take it when they are abed: let them lye upon their back &
> keep it in their mouth, till it is dissolved & so sleepe. If the mouth
> or throat be very Soare You may take Six penny weight.[60]

Lady Butler's honey is most likely local; the Bole Aremeniack, or more regularly bole Armoniac, is another matter. It is not just the product of a (usually) faraway land; it is earth itself. According to the *Oxford English Dictionary*, bole Armoniac is "soft friable fatty earth, usually of a pale red colour" named in English medicinal recipes as early as the fifteenth century;[61] in particular, it was valued for its astringent properties and perceived ability to fight plague and smallpox.[62] Usually, bole Armoniac was assumed to be imported from Armenia,[63] and indeed Galen connected it to the Armenian city of Bagawan in his discussion of the clay's power.[64] Listed among other drugs in the *Book*

60 Fanshawe, *Mrs. Fanshawe's Booke of Receipts*, 1678, Wellcome MS 7113, 32v.

61 "bole Armoniac" in "ammoniac, adj., sense 1.b," in *Oxford English Dictionary*, accessed July 18, 2023.

62 Galen notes that Armenian bole was used for "various kinds of stomach ailments, for mouth ulcers, and was administered to those suffering from breathing difficulties," as well as contagious diseases such as smallpox, adding that "Dioscorides described the so-called armenion as blue in colour." In a recent study, scientists examining six medicinal earths held at the Pharmacy Museum of the University of Basel tested their effectiveness on two pathogens. "Of the six, only one was found to be bioactive against both. This was the red earth 01405, which is presumed be an Armenian bole." See Danae Venieri et al., "Bridging the Gaps: Bole and Terra Sigillata as Artefacts, as Simples and as Antibacterial Clays," *Minerals* 10 (2020): 4, 7.

63 "Board nail–Bone comb," in Nancy Cox and Karin Dannehl, eds., *Dictionary of Traded Goods and Commodities 1550–1820* (Wolverhampton: University of Wolverhampton, 2007), *British History Online*, accessed September 17, 2019.

64 Venieri writes that, "Galen mentions that it originated in a mountain in the city of Bagouana which is a Hellenised rendering of the ancient Armenian Bagawan, a place that was most probably

of Rates, as "Bolus communis, or Armoniacus,"[65] the specific properties of this soil involve more than countering swelling and fever; their ingestion quite literally integrates the soil of a faraway place into the patient's body, linking her to an environment otherwise outside of her own experience. Lady Butler's treatment thus requires her patients to more than consume the fruits of foreign lands; they must incorporate the land itself.[66] In Stacy Alaimo's words, the clay "take[s] up residence" in the suffering person's body, implanting a bit of Armenian land into their otherwise bedridden flesh.[67]

Despite the geographic location embedded in its name, early modern writers associated the name *bole Armoniac* with other locations as well—among them, perhaps surprisingly, Virginia. As Danae Venieri argues, the process of loosening the link between the name of a medicinal clay and its point of origin began with Ottoman Empire's restrictions on the export of much-valued Lemnian earth from the island of Lemnos in the sixteenth century; this change in the market spurred the search for other sources of medicinal clay, boosting the reputations of earths ranging from Terra Sigillata (France), English boles, Earth of Ireland, as well as bole Armoniac—"all clearly denoting place of origin, albeit in very broad geographical terms."[68] Indeed, *The Rates of Merchandizes* includes both "Terra Lemnia" and "Terra Sigillata" in its tables, pointing to their use in English cures; these earths, however, were taxed by the pound, while bole Armoniac was taxed by the "hund[red] weight, cont. 112 [pounds]," suggesting it was more easily obtained.[69] Edward Chamberlayne's remark that "*Fullers Earth,* is no where else produced in that abundance and excellency as in *England*" praises locally sourced options for these ingredients as well.[70] Nonetheless, discussions of medicinal clay used these names interchangeably, often resulting in a geographical mishmash.

near today's Diyad in the Turkish Province of Ağrı, very close to the modern Turkish–Armenian border." Venieri et al., "Bridging the Gaps," 8.

65 *The Rates of Merchandizes*, 1642, 15; Anne Stobart also discusses the compound's importation; see Anne Stobart, *Household Medicine in Seventeenth-Century England* (London: Bloomsbury, 2016), 86.

66 The recipe in Fanshawe's manuscript undergoes a different sort of digestion, since it is crossed out, though it's not clear when or by whom. For more on these markings in recipe books, see Leong, *Recipes and Everyday Knowledge*, 112–18.

67 Alaimo, *Bodily Natures*, 102.

68 Venieri et al., "Bridging the Gaps," 2. For a comprehensive look at medicinal earths in early modern Europe, see Arthur MacGregor, "Medicinal terra sigillata: A Historical, Geographical and Typological Review," in *A History of Geology and Medicine,* eds. C. J. Duffin, R. T. J. Moody, and C. Gardner-Thorpe (London: London Geological Society, 2013), 113–36.

69 *The Rates of Merchandizes*, 1642, 21–22, 15.

70 Edward Chamberlayne, *Angliæ notitia, or The Present State of England Together with Divers Reflections upon the Antient State Thereof* (London, 1669), 11.

John Smith, for example, used all these designations and more to describe the soil along the Virginia coastline: "The colour of the earth we found in diverse places, resembleth *bole Armoniac, terra sigillata ad lemnia*, Fullers earth marle and divers other such appearances."[71] His note applies descriptions of soils specifically identified with Armenia, France, the isle of Lemnos, and England, to the so-called New World. Smith evidently carries within his bodily senses his experience of other soils, framing his observations of Virginia according to the lands he has encountered before. And he is not alone in doing so. Thomas Hariot also described a local medicinal soil, called *wapeih* in the local Algonquian language, as "very like to terra sigillata: and hauing beene refined, it hath beene found by some of our Phisitio[n]s and Chirurgeons to bee of the same kinde of vertue and more effectuall."[72]

The soils of Virginia, like that associated with Armenia and other geographical locations, could thus by their own powers cure English bodies. While an urge to gain market share may have motivated this blending of medicinal earths, the result nonetheless was an implied claim that these soils worked for all bodies. Given these well-touted curative powers, it only follows that merchants sought out these soils, and no wonder English people would swallow them whole.

Forever Rooted

Even as soil itself became more portable and less particular, Ann Fanshawe absorbed the special traits of lands she experienced, her travels infusing her body with the properties of these foreign places more deeply. By the time Fanshawe settled in Yorkshire, her body carried within it traces of London, Ireland, and Spain, not to mention waystations and ships she occupied along the way. The period of stillness and rest in Yorkshire allowed her to contemplate the travels and faraway places that took up residence within her. The Averie section of her recipe manuscript reflects her effort to consolidate her experiences and to form, with intention, connections to a new landscape and an expanding family.[73] Fanshawe's brief account of settling into Tankersley Park makes clear that she is putting down roots,

71 John Smith, *A Map of Virginia* (London, 1612), 3.

72 Thomas Hariot, *A Briefe and True Report of the New Found Land of Virginia* (London, 1590), 8.

73 Archer, "'An Offering to her Memory,'" 117–43. She offers a sense of the book's stages of composition, as well as family members, and notes that "This time [in Yorkshire] provided the Fanshawes, freed from the demands of political service, with a rare period of introspection," Archer, "'An Offering to her Memory,'" 130.

quite literally, while setting out to entwine herself with the people of the area. She notes that,

> In March we with our 3 children, Ann, Richard, and Betty, went into Yorkshire, where we livd an innocent country life, minding only the country sports and the country affairs. Here my husband translated Luis de Camoens, and in October the 8th, 1653, I was delivered of my daughter Margarett. I found all the nighbourhood very civil and kind upon all occasions, the place plentyfull and healthfull and very pleasant; but there was no fruit untill we planted some; and my Lord Straford says now that what we planted is the best fruit in the north.[74]

As David Goldstein notes, this passage reveals Fanshawe's attempt to become part of the area's "network of objects and people," efficiently embedding herself with the activities and inhabitants of the area. Fanshawe, "like fruit trees in an orchard," is "making her mark by becoming part of her world rather than separating herself from it."[75]

That world includes the soil of Tankersley Park, which permeates Fanshawe's being as much as her plantings affect the landscape. The place gets under her skin, becoming part of her physical and psychological makeup, refusing to let go even after she and her family leave Yorkshire in 1654. Immediately after her mention of planting fruit trees, Fanshawe moves into one of the memoir's most wrenching passages, recounting the death of her first daughter Ann:

> The house of Tankersly and parke are both very pleasant and good, and we livd there with great content. But God had ordered that it should not last, for upon the 20th of July, 1654, at 3 a clock in the afternoon, dyed our most dearly beloved daughter Ann Fanshawe, whose beauty and wit exceeded all that ever I saw of her age. She was between 9 and 10 years old, very tall, and the dear companion of our travells and sorrows; she lay sick but five dayes of the small pox, in which time she expressed so many wise and devout sayings as is a miracle from her years. We both wished to have gone into the grave with her. She lyes buryed in Tankersly Church, and her death made us both desirous to quit that fatall place to us.[76]

74 Fanshawe, *The Memoirs of Ann, Lady Fanshawe*, edited by Loftis, 136.

75 Goldstein, *Eating and Ethics*, 163.

76 Fanshawe, *The Memoirs of Ann, Lady Fanshawe*, edited by Loftis, 136.

Fanshawe jumps from orchard-planting at Tankersley to the death of her daughter—in a passage that begins with the matter-of-fact announcement of another daughter's birth at the same location. The conjunction of the park's budding potential for abundance, with newly planted trees and the happy, if not overtly celebrated, arrival of her new daughter Margaret, gives way to the sudden, comparatively detailed story of her daughter Ann's death after suffering "but five days of the small pox." Jarring as it may be, this juxtaposition of her Yorkshire home's initial fruitfulness with the acknowledgment of the staggering grief upon the death of their first child allows readers a glimpse of Fanshawe's interior world—something that many scholars have concluded is missing in her otherwise businesslike memoir.[77] She and her husband are overcome with the need to "quit that fatall place," but leaving Tankersley cannot excise Fanshawe's connection to its land. The place becomes a tender but essential element in her liveliness, in Alaimo's words "tak[ing] up residence within the body" with the painful memory of a daughter who "lies buried in Tankersly Church" near the thriving fruit trees she planted but never saw mature. In her early days in Yorkshire, Fanshawe seemed not to have imagined leaving either behind; while she might depart hastily to avoid the memories that haunt her there, Fanshawe cannot sever her connections to the land, even though she occupied it for such a brief time.

This attachment to Tankersley Park is particularly compelling given that Fanshawe suffers through the death of many other children. Mary Beth Rose argues that, even though Fanshawe "is almost constantly pregnant, miscarrying, or giving birth" during the events of her memoir, she "assigns a secondary value" to these experiences, and, as a result, "a crucial tale … remains untold, namely, the saga of Fanshawe's female body."[78] Fanshawe certainly distances herself from the births of her children, declaring "My dear husband had six sons and eight daughters, borne and christned" and adding "I miscarryed of 6 more" as if to take more direct responsibility for the pregnancies with unhappy endings. But her apparent stoniness gives way to a careful record of the locations where the children's bodies were buried at the end of their young lives.

> Harrison my eldest son, and Henry my second son, Richard my third, and Henery my fourth, and Richard my fifth are all dead. My third lyes

77 Fanshawe's memoir has often been called impersonal; Seelig says this quality stems from her mission to record the family's history, not her own. See Sharon Cadman Seelig, *Autobiography and Gender in Early Modern Literature: Reading Women's Lives, 1600–1680* (Cambridge: Cambridge University Press, 2006), 91.

78 Rose, *Gender and Heroism in Early Modern English Literature*, 70.

> buried in the Protestant Churchyard in Paris, by the father of the Earl of Bristol.
>
> My eldest daughter Ann lyes buried in the parish church of Tankersley in Yorkshire, where she dyed. Elizabeth lyes in the chappell of the French Hospitall at Madrid, where she dyed of a feavor at 10 days old. My next daughter of her name lyes buryed in the parish of Fotts Cray in Kent near Frogpool, my brother Warrick's house, where she dyed, and my fourth daughter Mary lies in my father's vault in Hartford with my first son Henry. My eldest lyes buried in the parish church of St. John's Colledge in Oxford, where he was born; my second Henry lyes in Bengey Church in Hartfordshire, and my second Richard in the Esperance in Lisbone in Portugall, he being borne 10 weeks before my time when I was in that court.[79]

Fanshawe's account traces her maternal mourning onto the map of her travels, marking out the ground where she has seen her children buried. She repeatedly returns to these deaths, recounting not just the facts of her children's brief lives but the places she gave birth to them and buried them. The above summary of her childbearing appears in the early pages of the memoir, attaching her children's names to the milestones on her journeys before offering detailed accounts of her adventures in these places. That is, she prepares readers to envision her children buried in Madrid, Lisbon, and Frogpool before knowing anything else about those places. Her phrasing—that the children "lye" in vaults and tombs—lends them an active power, keeping them in the present tense even after their bodily deaths. Each child is mentioned again in the text when the narrative reaches their dates of birth and death, and Fanshawe appends a second list of her children, complete with places of birth and death, to the memoir. Fanshawe thus sets out multiple frameworks for containing and sharing her grief, revisiting the locations and circumstances that shape her most personal maternal experiences. Madrid and Tankersley, in other words, become places of mourning, and the sorrow experienced there permeates and reshapes her body just as much as the food and medicine she ingests there.

The remedies Fanshawe records in her book, with their blend of imported ingredients and locally grown products, in turn have an impact on the bodies of Fanshawe's family members and friends. The salves, tonics, and pills that these recipes create allow different natural products to take up residence

79 Fanshawe, *The Memoirs of Ann, Lady Fanshawe*, edited by Loftis, 106–7.

in the patient's body. They take elements from far and wide and make them part of the individual, realigning balances in the body by embedding in it foreign materials that nudge the sufferer's physical constitution into a healthier state. In that sense, these imports alter the bodies they treat, reshaping their lived experiences, as well as their relationship to their surroundings. In Fanshawe's case, these recipes resonate in yet another way, awakening memories of family members, their sickness and suffering as well as their willingness to share knowledge. These memories may be suggested in her memoir, but the networks of meaning that create her family history are far more visible in her recipes. There, the impact of her father's work, her mother's experiences as a lively and experimental cook and caregiver, and her family's unarticulated connection to colonial concerns are made manifest on the page, alongside Fanshawe's efforts to merge her own experiences with those of her husband's kin. In this sense, her recipe book does more than traces social networks; it shows the extent to which the lands she and her family have experienced permeate their bodies, shaping their interactions with the present world and bearing the lingering, internalized physical residue of the places of their pasts. The memories of the people contributing to the recipe book may stay with her, but the recipes they create are part of her flesh, ministering to her present health while also influencing her bodily future.

4. Keeping English Bodies: Preserving, Seasoning, and Englishness in Early Virginia Recipes

Abstract: This chapter focuses on recipes for Dr. Stevens's Water, a home medicine purported to preserve bodies into extreme age, to explore the importance English settlers placed on bodily integrity when in unfamiliar territories. The realities of disease and hunger in colonial Virginia, however, forced the English to question their assumptions of longevity. The physical adjustments settlers underwent threatened to undermine both the ambitions of the new colony and the long-established humoral principles of *Airs, Waters, Places*. The recipe manuscripts kept by the Randolph family, however, rarely acknowledged these challenges, instead repeating standard, soothing recipes. The enduring appeal of inherited recipes revealed an adherence to nationalistic ideas of health and nutrition in a land full of strange plants and diseases.

Keywords: Dr. Stevens's Water; Gervase Markham; cannibalism; seasoning; humors; preservation

When Ann Fanshawe's uncle George Harrison arrived in Jamestown in 1619, the plantation had existed for just over a decade, struggling to survive on the Virginia coast. Since its founding in 1608, the settlement had experienced famine and disease, as well as unstable relationships with the area's Algonquian peoples. All the while, the Virginia Company kept an eye on the bottom line, insisting that the plantation turn a profit for its investors. This meant that the Company routinely reminded those who made the Atlantic crossing that their chief duty remained exporting goods for sale in England and Europe. Such intense focus on finding, securing, and (later) producing marketable commodities meant that, in the plantation's early years, the English at Jamestown envisioned Virginia as a temporary

Nunn, Hillary M. *Recipes on the Move in Early Modern England and British North America: Domestic Medicine, Mobility, and Manuscript Culture*. Amsterdam: Amsterdam University Press, 2025.
DOI 10.5117/9789463723398_CH04

settlement, a place to make fortunes rather than homes. In the words of a Virginia Company document dated July 16, 1621, "[T]he Mynds of our people in Virgenia are much dejected, and ther hartes enflamed with a desire to returne for England only through the wants of the comforts without which God saw that Man could not live contentedlie[,] noe not [even] in Paradize." Vehemently clinging to the long-advertised Edenic qualities of Virginia's lands, more than twenty investors pledged their financial support to a marriage scheme to make the tidewater plantation a bit homier:

> Wee therfore judginge itt a Christian charitie to releive the disconsolate mindes of our people ther, and a speciall advancement to the Plantation, to tye and roote the Planters myndes to Virginia by the bonds of wives and children: have resolved and doe by our hands hereunder binde our selves to paie into the handes of Master Thomas Gibbs [to send] of *young, handsome, and honestlie educated Maides* to Virginia: Ther *to be disposed in Marriage to the most honest and industrious Planters who shall defray and sattisfie* us *the Charges of their passages and provisions att such rates as they and* our *Agents shall agree.*[1]

Less than a month later, the Virginia Company outlined the process for pairing twelve women who agreed to make their homes in Jamestown with new husbands on the plantation. The Company's leaders did so in a letter dated August 12, 1621, which accompanied one widow and eleven maids on the *Marmaduke* bound for Virginia. Only the most prosperous men could successfully court the new arrivals, since earning the women's hands in marriage required a payment of 120 pounds of tobacco. But the letter also promised that "There are neare fiftie more [women] w[hich] are shortly to come." The investors, in other words, were determined to give the colony roots, reasoning that "the Plantac[i]on can never flourish till families be planted, and the respect of wiues and Children fix the people on the Soyle."[2]

The Virginia Company investors, in other words, considered the bodies of colonists—and of their hoped-for families—as the seeds of their expansion efforts. In their view, the only way that Jamestown could flourish was for its occupants to be more firmly planted in their American surroundings.

1 David R. Ransome "Wives for Virginia, 1621," *The William and Mary Quarterly* 48, no. 1 (1991): 7. Ransome reprints this document from the Ferrar Papers at Magdalene College, in Ransome "Wives for Virginia, 1621," 3–18.

2 Susan Myra Kingsbury ed., *The Records of the Virginia Company* (Washington, DC, 1906–35), 3:493.

Family trees, complete with American-born children of English blood, offered the best opportunity for creating a lasting connection between the colonists and the occupied land, forcing the English to see themselves as physically connected to, not just economically invested in, the surrounding environment. The plantation, in short, needed to be more fully anchored in American soil, and producing a new generation on and of Virginia was the best strategy for accomplishing this goal.

Rootedness in Virginia, however, suggested a disconnection from English soil, and such transplantation threatened not just to displace the settlers but to transform their bodies—and identities—from the inside out. As James Lind wrote roughly a century later, when settler colonialism had become firmly established as central to English commerce:

> Men who thus exchange their native for a distant climate, may be considered as affected in a manner somewhat analagous to that of plants, removed into a foreign soil; where the utmost care and attention are required, to keep them in health, and inure them to their new situation; since, thus transplanted, some change and alteration must happen in the constitutions of both.[3]

While taking for granted that the English abroad would alter the lands they occupied, Lind frankly admits that the climates would certainly change English bodies as well. Echoing the familiar Hippocratic ideas of *Airs, Waters, Places*, Lind outlines a process that had come to be known, in the early days of Virginia's colonization, as *seasoning*—that is, the experience of bodily illness brought on by the physical shock of immersion in an alien climate. Seasoning realigned the humors of colonizing bodies to their new surroundings after transplantation, and it signaled a potential shift in their cultural identity alongside this physical transition. In short, seasoning marked settlers in America as losing some of their Englishness—an idea that threatened the settlers' sense of national, biological, and racial identity even as it helped strengthen their connection to their new homes.

As early participants in England's colonial efforts, Jamestown's residents resisted these cultural and bodily changes, working to maintain what they saw as their physical differences from the Indigenous people they met in Virginia. Demanding English food and imported medicines, the colonists stubbornly insisted on their bodily need for familiar sustenance. Like the

3 James Lind, *An Essay on Diseases Incidental to Europeans in Hot Climates* (London, 1768), 2–3.

Spanish conquistadors Rebecca Earle examines, Jamestown's settlers were certain that "Food helped make them who they were in terms of both their character and their very corporeality, and it was food, more than anything else, that made European bodies different from Amerindian bodies."[4] Much to the Virginia settlers' surprise, the promised Edenic landscape did not produce familiar English crops, and colonists were left to struggle with the threat to their identity that came with raising and consuming native grains. How could new immigrants who ate like members of Virginia's Algonquian tribes, they wondered, keep from losing their English constitutions? If fed with American foods, at what point would their English bodies start to look, behave, and think like those of the people whose land they sought to exploit for economic gain? The resulting resistance to such permanent transplantation—encapsulated in the colonists' strenuous effort to preserve their bodily identity despite the Virginia environment—left the English largely dependent on goods brought by supply ships from the other side of the Atlantic, even when the land around them offered raw materials that could nurture their survival, as well as make them a profit.

This chapter concentrates on two recipes for bodily preservation associated with Virginia's earliest English settlers, using these very different texts to highlight the importance of maintaining English identity after transplantation to the American colony. The two recipes call on English domestic practices long established in manuscript collections and passed from generation to generation. The recipes share a concern for the importance of preserving not just English bodies but the medical and cultural knowledge conveyed in their words. "In recipes," Wendy Wall argues, "humans and edibles shared a structural place, as things in need of survival and duration," and the recipes themselves "reiterated and duplicated" materials in an act of textual preservation.[5] Though these recipes repeat drastically different cultural narratives, both work to reinforce concepts central to the notion of Englishness—notions that were in danger of erosion when living in lands where Indigenous bodies and practices enjoyed a more direct connection to the surrounding environments.

Virginia Company records show that the more complicated recipe—for the cure-all cordial known as Dr. Stevens's Water—appears in a printed

4 Rebecca Earle, *The Body of the Conquistador: Food, Race and the Colonial Experience in Spanish America, 1492–1700* (Cambridge: Cambridge University Press, 2012), 2.

5 Wendy Wall, *Recipes for Thought: Knowledge and Taste in the Early Modern Kitchen* (Philadelphia: University of Pennsylvania Press, 2015), 174, 168. Wall's chapter "Temporalities: Preservation, Seasoning, and Memorialization" offers a compelling look at preservation as healthcare, particularly in relation to Shakespeare's *All's Well That Ends Well.*

household guide shipped to the colony, Gervase Markham's *Countrey Contentments*. Firmly linked to English readers and locations, the recipe inscribes cultural and biological strength and tenacity, as well as communicates medical knowledge allegedly capable of prolonging life. Despite its complexity, the recipe for Dr. Stevens's Water, as we shall see, was itself something of a survivor, circulating in both print and manuscript in England and making its way into the collections of home practitioners in Virginia and neighboring colonies. The second recipe, by contrast, is prepared in secret and offered without explicit instruction. Rather than providing Virginia wives guidance in preserving life, this recipe results in a wife who is herself preserved—literally, in that her starving husband murders her and salts her body, as good housekeeping would demand, for later consumption. Framed as a tale of the colony's hardships, this recipe's explicit cannibalism nonetheless provides English food for English people, illustrating in its skewed domesticity the extremes to which early settlers would go to limit their bodily connections to Virginian products. The two recipes illustrate the pervasive re-inscription of English domestic practices of preservation— both of food and of bodily health—on American soil. At the same time, these two accounts of preservation techniques underscore how imported recipes themselves worked to capture and perpetuate English cultural identity, even in the most extreme situations. The endurance of the recipes in the region's manuscript collections testifies to the lasting power of domestic practice in defining and reinforcing settler cultural identity in contrast to Indigenous practices.

English Identity and Recipe Texts in Seventeenth-Century Virginia

The Englishwomen who arrived in Virginia on the *Marmaduke* were largely unprepared to establish homesteads in their unfamiliar surroundings. To be selected to make the journey, most had offered letters of recommendation to the Virginia Company that stressed moral character and good temperament rather than skills. As David R. Ransome shows, thirty-seven of the fifty-seven women arriving on two transports in 1621 were accustomed to a cosmopolitan life as residents of London, or at least carried the endorsement of relatives who lived in the city; in fact, by Ransome's count, "only one or two appear to have come up from the country to go to Virginia."[6]

6 Ransome, "Wives for Virginia, 1621," 12.

Only the two oldest women brought letters that hinted at preparation for homesteading. Alice Burges, 28, was "skillfull in anie countrie worke. She can brue, bake, and make malte &c," while Ann Tanner, at 26 or 27, could "Spinn and sewe in blackworke ... brue, and bake, make butter and cheese, and doe huswifery."[7] Scholars have generally assumed the remaining women had little preparation for the trials of plantation life, yet the scant nature of records leaves room to imagine some relevant experience. Ransome implies that eight other women's connections to landed gentry signaled their ignorance of rural housekeeping, despite the traditions of household management and medical care that drove the compilation of the recipe manuscripts found among landed families.[8] Similarly, even though many of the women where connected to London, Company records trace some of their births to places like Yorkshire and Gloucestershire, where they could have easily have gained experience with rural household work.[9]

Ransome's analysis of the possessions Jamestown brides brought with them from England makes no notes of manuscript recipe books, and little indication of such collections in early Virginia survives—that is, if such books existed in the early colony at all. The extreme conditions of colonial life, after all, would work against the preservation of such collections. In the colonies, these manuscripts could easily be damaged or abandoned, and they may not have made their way to new owners after their compilers' unexpected deaths. Nonetheless, by the end of the seventeenth century, many wills and inventories reveal that some individuals—including women like Sarah Willoughby—had substantial collections of books,[10] and that some women gifted books to other women.[11] Further into the seventeenth century, traces of recipe manuscripts in Virginia emerge, suggesting that the tradition of keeping

7 Ransome, "Wives for Virginia, 1621," 15.

8 Ransome, "Wives for Virginia, 1621," 12.

9 Jennifer Potter, *The Jamestown Brides: The Story of England's Maids for Virginia* (Oxford: Oxford University Press, 2019), 311–18.

10 Edward W. James, "Libraries in Colonial Virginia," *The William and Mary Quarterly* 3, no. 1 (1894): 44.

11 David D. Hall, "The Chesapeake in the Seventeenth Century," in *A History of the Book in America: Vol. 1: The Colonial Book in the Atlantic World,* eds. Hugh Amory and David D. Hall (Chapel Hill: University of North Carolina Press, 2007), 70. Hall further points out that household inventories in Virginia's York County describe not just books but "writings" and papers, usually stored in chests or trunks. The "sheer mass of written documents that both women and men handled in making property transactions," Hall concludes, suggests that "most of them had some capacity as readers." See Hall, "The Chesapeake in the Seventeenth Century," 70. Though Hall assumes that most of these handwritten papers were business documents, such collections of paper could easily offer traces of domestic accounts and household recipes.

such household collections had been in practice there all along. Kevin J. Hayes names several existing recipe books associated with the women of George Washington's plantation in Mount Vernon; he also points out that Virginia housekeepers wrote their own recipes into printed volumes already present in their kitchen.[12] Manuscripts kept and shared among family members also began to become visible in the records, among them the recipe collections kept by the Randolph family, to be discussed in this chapter.

While these later compilations may not date to the founding of Jamestown, they provide insight into the practices that took hold in the colony's earliest days. As is common with manuscript recipe collections, the techniques and treatments in these colonial books harken back generations, recording cures and culinary dishes common in England, sometimes with attribution but other times without any explicit attempt to outline a practice's origin. Thus, even eighteenth-century manuscript recipe collections, begun by families that transplanted themselves to Virginia, contain and build upon recipes originally meant to be useful in England but brought to America, alongside those modified, learned, or improvised in the colonies. Notably, these collections rarely attribute recipes to members of Indigenous tribes, let alone name individuals who conferred their knowledge on English settlers, though such transfers clearly took place. These colonial manuscript recipe collections took part in obscuring Indigenous knowledge, implicating their compilers in the archival violence associated with other, more commonly recognized means of eliminating traces of earlier cultures.[13]

With or without the help of recipe books, Englishwomen had been a key part of healthcare efforts in Jamestown for over a decade by the time the *Marmaduke* arrived. The colony's few Englishwomen oversaw the lodging, feeding, and nursing of single men, often taking in dying colonists who remembered these ministrations in their wills.[14] In fact, Thomas Niccolls argued that one of the reasons the colony needed more women was because so many of the men there "dye miserablie through nastines & many dep[ar]te the World in their owne dung for want of help in their sickness."[15] The

12 Kevin J. Hayes, *A Colonial Woman's Bookshelf* (Knoxville: University of Tennessee Press, 1996), 87–88.

13 For a discussion of this archival violence, see the Introduction and Jennifer Park, "Teaching Recipes, Race, and Erasure in the Early Modern Classroom," *Studies in Medieval and Renaissance Teaching* 28, no. 2 (2021): 61–79.

14 H. R. McIlwaine, *Minutes of the Council and General Court of Colonial Virginia, 1622–32, 1670–76* (Richmond: The Colonial Press, 1924), 50, 130.

15 Kingsbury, *Records of the Virginia Company*, 4:231. Chaplin also cites Niccolls to highlight the need for nurses in the colony. See Joyce E. Chaplin, *Subject Matter: Technology, the Body, and*

women's efforts enabled the colony to survive the Starving Time, the winter of 1609–10, when Virginia lacked English medical professionals.[16] While the Company had in its earliest days sent two doctors to Jamestown, as well as several apothecaries, these trained medical men could not adequately tend to the plantation's many sick and injured Englishmen. The apothecaries were charged chiefly with assessing American plants, and the cures made from them, as possible sources of profit. Some doctors shared this interest, as the physician John Clayton's writings about Algonquian cures show, yet many were simply overwhelmed with their duties, and they in turn were susceptible to the illness and starvation marking the colony's first years.[17]

Scholars have largely interpreted the domestic skills of the colony's early women as deficient, aligning their meagre abilities with those of the Jamestown men who struggled to cultivate crops for both survival and export. "Like Jamestown's early gentlemen," Hayes writes, these women "lacked practical, everyday survival skills. Books, they realized, contained information necessary to help them stay alive and healthy."[18] When they demanded help from the Company, Richard Berkeley and John Smith sent assistance by way of a ship aptly named the *Supply* in 1620, in the form of "Markhams and Goovges booke of all kind of English husbandry and huswifry and .2 others for the ordering of silk and silkworms."[19] Significantly, agricultural practices for profit and trade, rather than for immediate household benefit, constitutes the main focus on these books—with texts on the theoretically money-making silk production constituting half of this little library.[20] Barnaby Googe's 1614 book *The Whole Art and Trade of Husbandry*, moreover, makes little gesture toward the work of housewifery.[21] Markham's books were another matter.

Science on the Anglo-American Frontier, 1500–1676 (Cambridge, MA: Harvard University Press, 2003), 181–82. For more on women as caregivers in Virginia, see Wyndham Bolling Blanton, *Medicine in Virginia in the Seventeenth-Century* (New York: Arno Press, 1972), 158–75.

16 See Virginia Bernhard, "Men, Women and Children at Jamestown: Population and Gender in Early Virginia, 1607–1610," *Journal of Southern History* 58, no. 4 (1992): 599–618.

17 See John Clayton, *The Reverend John Clayton: A Parson with a Scientific Mind*, eds. Edmund Berkely and Dorothy Smith Berkeley (Charlottesville: Virginia Historical Society, 1965), discussed in chapter 5.

18 Hayes, *A Colonial Woman's Bookshelf*, 80.

19 Kingsbury, *The Records of the Virginia Company*, 3:400.

20 Powell notes that one of the silkworm books was probably *Observations to Be Followed, For the Making of Fit Roomes to Keepe Silk-Wormes In*. See William S. Powell, "Books in the Virginia Colony before 1624," *The William and Mary Quarterly* 5, no. 2 (1948): 180.

21 Other best-selling practical treatises arrived in Virginia in the first half of the seventeenth century, including the midwifery text *The Birth of Mankynd*, and one of Markham's chief sources, Charles Estienne's *Maison Rustique or The Country Farme*. The usefulness of these imported

Of the books on the *Supply*, Gervase Markham's have earned the most attention, largely because of his popularity in early modern England. His numerous how-to treatises on rural life offered domestic help in many forms and under many titles, and they were bound together in different combinations. His most substantial advice on housekeeping appearing in *The English Husvvife*, which appeared bound within the same volume as the 1615 *Countrey Contentments. The English Husvvife* focuses on establishing smoothly running households and is itself split into two parts: cooking and preserving food and preparing and administering medicines to the sick. Wendy Wall argues that Markham's domestic manuals were instrumental in creating, or at least reinforcing, ideas of Englishness, making their arrival in Virginia resonate with nationalistic importance.[22] This Englishness, however, worked against the books' usefulness. Jennifer Mylander points out that, as "steady sellers," Markham's books brought a familiar Englishness with them to American shores; the advice they offered, however, proved far from practical, assuming "an English environment in land and climate and an English culture in terms of commodities and labor."[23] Markham's perpetuation of ideas of English self-sufficiency nonetheless held appeal for Jamestown's transplanted population, who aimed to, in Mylander's words, render Virginia "more productive through the use of English practices, suggest[ing] that the land will be made more English as well."[24]

books sometimes declined upon arrival. Quinn notes that the medical advice in Philip Barough's *Method of Physicke* "is likely to have been more misleading than helpful to settlers who were trying to acclimatize themselves to American conditions and doing so unsuccessfully in the face of heavy mortality from diseases for whose effects textbooks such as this offered little remedy." See James, "Libraries in Colonial Virginia," 44 and David B. Quinn, "A List of Books Purchased for the Virginia Company," *The Virginia Magazine of History and Biography* 77, no. 3 (1969): 357. For further detail about books available in the colonies in the second half of the seventeenth century, see Hayes, *A Colonial Woman's Bookshelf*, 80–100. Meanwhile, Mylander offers a sustained look at Culpeper's importance to English colonial medicine. See Jennifer Mylander, "Early Modern 'How-To' Books: Impractical Manuals and the Construction of Englishness in the Atlantic World," *Journal for Early Modern Cultural Studies* 9, no. 1 (2009): 133–38. But some texts that traveled to Virginia, like Gerard's *Herball*, at least attempted to incorporate knowledge of American ingredients and environments, filtered as it was through the eyes of earlier European visitors to the continent and experiments conducted on the eastern side of the Atlantic. See Powell, "Books in the Virginia Colony before 1624," 181.

22 See Wall for the many combinations of Markham's treatises in bound books. Mylander and Powell discuss Markham's books but do not speculate as to which ones would have made this journey. See Mylander, "Early Modern 'How-To' Books," 123–24; Powell, "Books in the Virginia Colony before 1624," 179; and Wendy Wall, *Staging Domesticity: Household Work and English Identity in Early Modern Drama* (Cambridge: Cambridge University Press, 2002), 37–40.

23 Mylander, "Early Modern 'How-To' Books," 124, 129.

24 Mylander, "Early Modern 'How-To' Books," 125.

When Markham's books arrived, the women of Jamestown would have read that their work involved, at its core, preservation; in undertaking this work, however, the women were in fact engaged in not just maintaining Englishness but helping it to take root in American soil. The English housewife, Markham explained, should devote herself to the "preseruation and care of the family"; she should know "how to administer many wholesome receits or medicines for the good of their healthes, as well to preuent the first occasion of sicknesse."[25] And to help do so, he aimed to keep his book simple, describing actions to restore family members to health rather than burden readers with explanations as to why they became ill in the first place. In doing so, he hoped to tightly circumscribe the housewife's duties to limit the complexity—and economic precarity—of her home. As noted in chapter 2, Markham links domesticity to Englishness itself when he decrees the proper housewife should work "with the prouisione of her owne yarde" rather than materials originating "from other Countries."[26] But these instructions put the English in Jamestown in an impossible position—they had already moved beyond England to their "own" faraway homesteads across the ocean. Their situation illustrates Amy Kaplan's observation that domesticity is "more mobile and less stabilizing" than typically recognized. Because it is involved in imperial expansion even as it serves as an anchor for settlers, domesticity "travels in contradictory circuits both to expand and contract the boundaries of home and nation and to produce shifting conceptions of the foreign."[27] And indeed Markham's books facilitated the perpetuation of English methods in the colony, helping housewives, themselves transplants, to establish traditional practices in their new homeland. When he implored his reader to make "her circle raither straight then large," Markham asked her to cordon off only the domain that she could successfully control. This cautious approach was for him an essentially defensive move, for, he reasons, "if we extend to the vttermost we take away increase ...: but if we preserue any part, we build strong forts against the aduersaries of fortune, prouided that such preseruation be honest and conscionable ...."[28]

Markham's advice for the preservation of health takes a prominent position in the book, though its concentration on English maladies in English environments offers little help to those struggling to adjust to Virginia's

25 Gervaise Markham, *Countrey Contentments, or The English husvvife* (London, 1615), 4.

26 Markham, *Countrey Contentments, or The English husvvife*, 4; this is also quoted in Wall, *Staging Domesticity*, 40.

27 Amy Kaplan, "Manifest Domesticity," *American Literature* 70, no. 3 (1998): 583.

28 Markham, *Countrey Contentments, or The English Husvvife*, 3.

climate. Instead, *The English Husvvife* records well-worn cures for ailments ranging from apoplexy to pimples. He offers some guidance for the most pressing condition Virginians encountered—the fevers that accompanied seasoning—but he admits that those fevers "comming from consumptions, and other long continued sicknesses, doe altogether surpasse our Hus-wiues capacity."[29] Aside from endorsing ale concoctions and nosegays to "preserue you from infection,"[30] few recipes deal with avoiding disease, instead working to stay the damage of illnesses after they arise. Preventing decay lies outside Markham's purview, though he does include a scant number of recipes for fruit conserves, butter, and cheeses designed to prolong food's usable life.[31] On the whole, Markham largely avoids the business of complicated formulas for overtly medical treatment. That is, with the exception of one remarkable recipe: Dr. Stevens's Water.

Dr. Stevens's Water and the Preservation of English Life

A medicine appearing over and over in English recipe books, both in print and manuscript, Dr. Stevens's Water typically calls for more than a dozen ingredients and makes grand promises not just for restoring health but preserving it into advanced age. While it has been suggested that Dr. Stevens was in fact the French doctor Charles Estienne, the identity of Dr. Stevens, or sometimes Stephens, remains largely a mystery[32]—so much so that

29 Markham, *Countrey Contentments, or The English Husvvife*, 5.

30 Markham, *Countrey Contentments, or The English Husvvife*, 86.

31 While he offers guidance for "the poudring up or potting of butter" and for making cheeses that will keep "a full yeere before you vse them," Markham offers only basic instruction for conserving fruit. See Markham, *Countrey Contentments, or The English Husvvife*, 113, 115. Aside from a trio of marmalade recipes, he includes only one general entry for preserving any other fruit, helpfully labeled "To make any conserue." Markham, *Countrey Contentments, or The English Husvvife*, 71, 78, 77.

32 Vincent DiMarco and Ken Albala link the water to the early sixteenth-century French physician Charles Estienne, and indeed the English translation of Estienne's work contains a similar water; Estienne's life, however, does not match the claims of longevity attached to some instances of the recipe. DiMarco makes this connection to Estienne in DiMarco, *It Has Helped to Admiration: Eighteenth-Century Medical Cures from the Kitchen Book of Bridget Lane* (Bloomington, IN: iUniverse, 2010), 38–40. DiMarco's book features a version of the water from Lane's text; see Bridget Lane, *Cookery and Medical Remedy Book*, 1737, Clark MS 2015.002, Clark Memorial Library, Los Angeles, CA, 19r–19v (the Clark Memorial Library catalog entry lists DiMarco as the former owner of that manuscript. See https://calisphere.org/item/ark:/21198/n15021/). Albala later asserts that the water "ultimately comes from Charles Estienne in the early sixteenth century"; see Ken Albala, "Stimulants and Intoxicants in Europe, 1500–1700," in *The*

Michelle DiMeo cites him as evidence that named recipes do not always signify a personal relationship between manuscript compilers and their cited sources.[33] The recipe had already enjoyed a long history in England before Markham published it, appearing in printed books in the late sixteenth century, and Karen Hess points out the recipe's endurance among early American collectors, calling it "the Bayer's aspirin of its day."[34] Scholars have helped keep this recipe alive, too, by calling on its various, and varying, appearances. To illustrate the interplay between print and manuscripts, for example, Jonathan Sanderson compares a Dr. Stevens's Water recipe in Diana Astry's seventeenth-century recipe book to a version in Culpeper's *Pharmacopoeia*.[35] Similarly, Katherine Knight connects the versions of Dr.

Routledge History of Food, ed. C. Helstosky (London: Routledge, 2014), 48, and John French, *The Art of Distillation* (London, 1651), 48. Given the claims associated with Dr. Stevens's Water, it is interesting to note the Estienne lived to the age of sixty (1504–64). See Konstantinos Markatos et al., "Charles Estienne (1504–1564): His Life, Work, and Contribution to Anatomy and the First Description of the Canal in the Spinal Cord," *World Neurosurgery* 100 (2017): 186.

33 Michelle DiMeo, "Authorship and Medical Networks: Reading Attributions in Early Modern Manuscript Recipe Books," in *Reading and Writing Recipe Books, 1550–1800,* eds. Michelle DiMeo and Sara Pennell (Manchester: Manchester University Press, 2013), 27. She also cites an example of Dr. Stevens's Water from Johanna St. John's manuscript. See DiMeo, "Authorship and Medical Networks," 43 n. 10 and Johanna St. John, *Johanna St. John her Book,* 1680, Wellcome MS 4338, Wellcome Collection, London, England, 29r.

34 As Hess notes, the recipes for Dr. Stevens's Water resemble Markham's in Thomas Cogan's *The Haven of Health* (London, 1636), 230–32; and Thomas Dawson, *The Good Husvvifes Ievvell,* (London, 1587), 39v–40r. See Karen Hess, ed., *Martha Washington's Booke of Cookery* (New York: Columbia, 1981), 404, 454.

35 While those two versions clearly resemble one another, they vary considerably from the version Markham records, in that neither describes the "preservative" nature of the medicine. Sanderson surveys instances of Dr. Stevens's Water in St. John's manuscript as well as Lady Barrett, *Select Receipts,* 1711, Wellcome MS 1071, Wellcome Collection, London, England, 38; he also reports finding the recipe in printed titles, M. B., *The Ladies Cabinet Enlarged and Opened* (London, 1654), 47–48, and Hugh Plat, *Delightes for Ladies* (London, 1602), E4v. See Jonathan Sanderson, "Nicholas Culpeper and the Book Trade: Print and the Promotion of Vernacular Medical Knowledge" (PhD dissertation, University of Leeds, 1999), 242 n. 153. Stitt compares Culpeper to Diana Astry in A. F. Cirket and Bette Stitt, eds. *English Wills, 1498–1526; Diana Astry's Recipe Book c. 1700* (London: Boydell & Brewer, 1957), 83–168. Fanshawe's manuscript contains a recipe for Dr. Stevens's Water, and her version stresses the cordial's preservative nature, as does Lady Carteret's version. See Ann Fanshawe, *Mrs. Fanshawes Book of Receipts,* 1678, Wellcome MS 7113, Wellcome Collection, London, England, 80r–80v and Grace Carteret, *Manuscript Recipe book of Grace Carteret, 1st Countess Granville,* 1654–1744, Wellcome MS. 8903, Wellcome Collection, London, England, 77r–77v. Lisa Smith mentions an occurrence of Dr. Stevens's Water in Bridget Hyde, *Madam Bridget Hyde her Receipt Book August the 19th Anno Domini 1676,* 1676–90, Wellcome MS 2990, Wellcome Collection, London, England, 52v in Lisa Smith, "Medicinal Compounds, Efficacious in Every Case," *The Recipes Project,* January 30, 2013. Anne Stobart describes four versions of Dr. Stevens's Water in Margaret Boscawen, Devon Heritage Center 1262M/FC /8, 200

Stevens's Water appearing in Lady Barrett's mid-seventeenth-century manuscript to Markham's print book.[36] The near omnipresence of Dr. Stevens's Water helps Elizabeth Spiller show that books of secrets could indeed have popular recipes in them[37] and leads Wendy Wall to compare the cordial to both Geritol and aspirin, suggesting its role as a mundane cure despite the complications in assembling and distilling its many ingredients.[38]

Recipe compilers often copied the many steps involved in making Dr. Stevens's Water into their manuscripts from print sources, and Markham's recipe makes its way almost verbatim into several Virginia manuscripts by the late seventeenth century. These versions of Dr. Stevens's Water bring with them English ideas of what is local, as well as of what is particularly English in the bodies under treatment. Markham's version is formatted as a prose paragraph without a heading, with its opening sentence immediately labeling the recipe and declaring its English character: "To make that soueraine water which was first inuented by Doctor *Steuens*, in the same forme as he deliuered the Receite to the Arch-bishop of *Canturbury*, a little before the death of the said Doctor." While Dr. Stevens's identity remains uncertain (and possibly French), his cure's link to the head of the Church of England anchors it firmly to an essentialized national identity. Such a direct connection proves all the more remarkable given that its first ingredient—the one required in greatest quantity—depends on a European source:

> Take a gallon of good Gaskoine wine, then take Ginger, Galuingale, Synamon, Nutmegges, Graines, Cloues bruised, Fennell seede, Carrawaie seede, Origanum; of euery of them a like quantitie, that is to say a dramme: then take Sage, wild Margerum, Peny-royall, Mints, Red-roses, Time, Pellitory, Rosemary, wild-time, Cammomill, Lauender, of each of them one handfull: then braie the spices small, and bruise the hearbes and put all into the

Recipes, Boscawen, 1668–87. See Anne Stobart, *Household Medicine in Seventeenth-Century England* (London: Bloomsbury, 2016), 40.

36 See Katherine Knight, "A Precious Medicine: Tradition and Magic in Some Seventeenth-Century Household Remedies," *Folklore* 113, no. 2 (2002): 239. Knight cites Barrett's manuscript, Egerton MS 1071.

37 Elizabeth Spiller, *Seventeenth-Century English Recipe Books: Cooking, Physic and Chirurgery in the Works of Elizabeth Talbot Grey and Aletheia Talbot Howard* (Burlington: Ashgate, 2011), xv–xvi.

38 Wall, *Recipes for Thought*, 173, 125. By 1655, Dr. Stevens's Water appears to be available commercially; a reference to the water, traded in gallons, appears in Nancy Cox and Karin Dannehl, eds., "Dr stephens water [*sic*]," *Dictionary of Traded Goods and Commodities 1550–1820* (Wolverhampton: University of Wolverhampton, 2007), *British History Online*, accessed September 17, 2019.

> wine, and let it stand so 12 houres, only stirre it diuers times, then distill it by a Limbecke, and keepe the first water by it selfe for that is the best, then keepe the second water for that is good, and for the last neglect it not, for it is very wholesom though the worst of the three.[39]

Beginning with wine from Gascony, in what is now southwest France, the recipe immediately demands ingredients from well beyond the English or the Virginian housewife's yard; the same can be said regarding many of the spices that make up the recipe's second step, particularly cinnamon, nutmeg, galangal, grains of paradise, ginger, and cloves. Gascoyne wine was so commonly used in England, however, that it may have begun to seem local, and the imported spices may have mingled long enough with locally grown oregano in the grocers' stalls that they no longer seemed exotic. Nonetheless, these spices were not generally plants that could be found in area fields—like the herbs in the second grouping, which could be gathered by the "handfull"—rather than measured out, in drammes, at a local shop. Still, many of the ingredients grew locally in England and were gathered using common knowledge of their habitats,[40] giving a distinct English flavor to the resulting distillation, and rendering a powerful effect on English bodies.

Markham next provides a long list of virtues associated with this water, ranging from the general (it "helpeth all inward diseases that commeth of cold") to the particular ("it is good against the shaking of the palsey," "cureth the contraction of sinnewes," "killeth the wormes," and "helpeth the conception of women that be barraine," among other things). But, most remarkably, Markham claims that Dr. Stevens's Water preserves life itself:

> [W]hosoeuer vseth this water moderately and not too often, preserueth him in good liking, and will make him seeme young in old age. With this water Docter *Steuens* preserued his owne life vntill such extreame age, that he could neither goe nor ride, and he continued his life being bed-rid fiue yeeres, when other Physicions did iudge hee could not liue one yeere, which he did confesse a little before his death; saying: that if he were sicke at anie time, he neuer vsed any thing but this water only...[41]

39 Markham, *Countrey Contentments or The English Husvvife*, 29.

40 For more on the different sorts of knowledge required in distillation and other preserving recipes, see Lucy J. Havard, "Preserve or Perish: Food Preservation Practices in the Early Modern Kitchen," *Notes and Records* 74 (2020): 5–33.

41 Markham, *Countrey Contentments or The English Husvvife*, 29–30.

Dr. Stevens's Water may in fact work too well, preserving Dr. Stevens himself for five bedridden years beyond his caretaker's prediction of his death. His use of his own water must have exceeded the moderate rate that the recipe says would make one "seeme young in olde age," instead leaving him immobile—"preserued" —in "extreame age." Withering in his bed, Dr. Stevens comes to resemble a living corpse, one that has undergone preserving treatment, more like a seasonal fruit or meat after annual slaughter than a human being.

Indeed, the recipe's narrative describes Dr. Stevens as preserved beyond the state that Markham, and other recipe writers, seem to find appropriate or appealing. Many later versions of the recipe make room for even further discomfort, extending their descriptions of Dr. Stevens to challenge the value of his ever-increasing longevity. For example, the recipe as recorded in Catherine Bacon's England-based manuscript claims Dr. Stevens lived to be "A hundred years lacking two & ten of | them he did live bedred";[42] Cogan's version in *The Haven of Health* also has Stevens living to 98, but he testifies that a full "twentie he lived bedred."[43] This depiction of the value of preserving life extends beyond Dr. Stevens in these accounts as well; the narrative concludes with his passing the recipe on to the Archbishop of Canterbury who, Markham tells us, "vsed it, and found such goodnesse in it that he liued till he was not able to drink of a cup, but sucked his drink through a hollow pipe of siluer."[44]

Even if Markham's narrative stretches credulity, it sets high expectations—not just for the cordial water's powers, but for the patients and caregivers who use it. English bodies with access to such a cordial should prove capable of extraordinarily long lives, and they should pass along both their physical longevity, and the medical skills that encourage it, to their English brethren. For colonists reading Markham's book, such extreme expectations not only reinforced the exceptional nature of their English roots, but also the cultural burden accompanying the process of transplanting themselves in territories abroad. Even if the colonists could survive and pass on their knowledge in their challenging American environment, could they do so with their foundational, supposedly enduring Englishness intact? Would access to Dr. Stevens's Water help?

42 Catherine Bacon, *Receipt Book of Catherine Bacon*, ca. 1680–1739, Folger V.a. 621, Folger Shakespeare Library, Washington, DC, 11.

43 Cogan, *The Haven of Health*, 231. M. B. claims that Stevens lived to the age of ninety-eight in M. B., *The Ladies Cabinet Enlarged and Opened*, 48.

44 Markham, *Countrey Contentments or The English Husvvife*, 30.

Seasoning and Preservation: Keeping English Bodies in Virginia

The survival of Dr. Stevens's Water in North American manuscripts is notable, given its lack of practicality in a struggling colonial setting. The new colony, after all, was no place for a bedridden elderly person unable to contribute to the settlement's work. But the bodily preservation that Dr. Stevens's Water promised kept alive an ideal of English identity threatened in Virginia's environment. The recipe emphasized not just the importance of English medicines concocted from (at least partially) English ingredients; it also reminded its readers of the English authorities—both religious and medical—who helped crystalize their English identities, creating a source of comfort, and duty, in strange surroundings. The recipe reminded the English settlers, in other words, of the humoral connections that still bound them to their homeland, even if their very survival in Virginia suggested those ties had loosened.

In recruiting colonists, the Virginia Company and the popular press painted the environment of the Jamestown settlement as Edenic and ideally suited to English bodies,[45] but the lived experience of the Chesapeake challenged that image of perfection. Despite the fact that Jamestown occupied a similar latitude to Spain, its weather was far from mild;[46] its summers were longer and its winters were far more bitter. Commentators noted that diseases in the Americas were in fact different from those found in similar settings in Europe, but such observations prompted adjustment to, rather than abandonment of, the *Airs, Waters, Places* ideas that drove much of the era's thinking about health. While the Hippocratic tradition "suggested that different diseases were to be found in different climates," Suman Seth notes that there remained "considerable disagreement over whether climates in very different geographical locations were, in fact, radically distinct."[47] To admit that these alien climates existed, and that these climates did not suit all human bodies equally, would be to admit that English settlers were not naturally suited or even adaptable to the land—that they were, in Seth's words, doomed to be fundamentally "out of place"[48] —and that their colonial project violated a sense of global, if not

45 For examples, see Chaplin, *Subject Matter*, 134; Suman Seth, *Difference and Disease: Medicine, Race, and the Eighteenth-Century British Empire* (Cambridge: Cambridge University Press, 2018), 40; and Alan S. Rome, *The English Embrace of the American Indians: Ideas of Humanity in Early America* (New York: Palgrave, 2017), 106.

46 Karen Ordahl Kupperman, "The Puzzle of the American Climate in the Early Colonial Period," *The American Historical Review* 87, no. 5 (1982): 1262–82.

47 Seth, *Difference and Disease*, 40.

48 Seth, *Difference and Disease*, 93.

divine, order. Rather than consider such a fundamental shift in thinking, English writers increasingly emphasized the ways that English bodies had come to thrive in the unfamiliar climate of the Americas after the initial, often lethal illnesses that came to be known as seasoning.

The notion of seasoning developed alongside colonization to resolve the conundrum of geographical and bodily specifics, providing a conceptual framework to trace the body's realignment to unfamiliar climates. According to Joyce E. Chaplin, the term *seasoning* was applied as far back to the 1550s to physical effects that Europeans in the Western hemisphere suffered from travel, when it was used to describe "adaptation to American air, sustenance, and diseases."[49] In Seth's words, seasoning is a "disease of *place*," one that affected only "those habituated to one location who ventured to another in which they were strangers."[50] In typical cases, seasoning marked a dangerous but concentrated time, sometimes defined as weeks or months or even years, during which newly arrived bodies suffered symptoms that could include fevers (yellow and malarial), dysentery, and other afflictions. Naturally, the condition required treatments derived from the environment that initially provoked the illness. Virginia governor Robert Beverley writes of new English settlers, "their Agues, are very troublesome, if a fit Remedy be not apply'd; but of late the Doctors there have made use of *Cortext Peruviana* [Peruvian bark] with Success, and find that it seldom or never fails to remove the Fits."[51] Though usually a temporary affliction, Beverley noted, some could suffer long-term effects from seasoning, becoming "over-run with obstinate scorbutick Humours" able to cause permanent damage,[52] in the form of rheumatic conditions that will be more thoroughly explored in the following chapter.

With its predictable harm to newly arrived bodies, the experience of seasoning was a shared one even though it might manifest differently in individual cases. As Seth puts it, "Seasoning presumed that all bodies were fundamentally the same: they merely had different histories," arriving with different humoral balances and thus different starting points for their period of adjustment.[53] This process insisted that human bodies themselves

49 Chaplin, *Subject Matter*, 151–52.

50 Seth, *Difference and Disease*, 93.

51 Robert Beverley, *The History and Present State of Virginia: A New Edition with an Introduction by Susan Scott Parish*, ed. Susan Scott Parish (Chapel Hill: University of North Carolina Press, 2013), 242.

52 Beverley, *The History and Present State of Virginia*, 243.

53 Suman Seth, "Race, Seasoning, and Strangeness: The Problem of Mobility in Early Modern Science and Medicine," *Global Intellectual History* 8, no. 4 (2022): 457.

were, in Chaplin's words, "natural products ... like trees felled in the old world, shipped like so much lumber to America, then dried, hardened, and proved durable in a new climate."[54] She posits English bodies as biological construction material, wood to be used in the building of a new Empire that these settlers in turn supported on their sturdy shoulders. And the timing of the process mattered as well. Ideally, settlers arrived in the fall or winter to avoid immediately confronting the diseases of Virginia's warm spring and summer. John Pory, the Colony secretary, bemoaned that warmer seasons were "fatall and unproffitable to new Comers," and that because they "Came in sickly," they could not do the "plantinge, settinge, howinge, clearinge ground, or buyldinge" so necessary at that time of year.[55] As the importation of enslaved African people to English colonies expanded after 1619, seasoning acquired new meanings, coming to refer not just to sickness prompted by new environment but to a process of brutal physical and psychological treatment at the hands of whites. This sometimes years-long "carefully designed management regime" forced Africans to adjust to American plantation procedures.[56] Seasoning, in short, altered all English bodies to fit their new American environment, but only enslaved Africans endured a purposefully scripted process at the hands of other humans in the colonies.[57]

But seasoning can be taken another way in the period: it can describe the processing of food to make it more suitable for individual tastes and—importantly—longer lasting. In the early modern period, the seasoning of food was about more than flavor; it was about modifying foods to render them more digestible and physically healthful. Seasonings customized food for the eater's body, tempering the innately cold or hot qualities of meals to achieve balance within those doing the consuming. Culinary seasoning, in this sense, gradually aligned human bodies with the surrounding

54 Chaplin, *Subject Matter*, 151.

55 Potter, *The Jamestown Brides*, 132–33.

56 See Nicholas Radburn, "'[M]anaged at First as if They Were Beasts': The Seasoning of Enslaved Africans in Eighteenth-Century Jamaica," *Journal of Global Slavery* 6, no. 1 (2021): 14. For a study of the medical aspects of this seasoning, see Sean Morey Smith, "Seasoning and Abolition: Humoral Medicine in the Eighteenth-Century British Atlantic," *Slavery and Abolition* 36, no. 4 (2015): 684–703.

57 As Lind reports, however, the Portuguese attempted to hurry seasoning in Africa, with disastrous results. Believing that the blood of those who survived relocation had been entirely replaced in the new climate, the Portuguese adopted a "most fatal method of seasoning people": "They, by small quantities, frequently repeated, took away as much blood as they supposed to be contained in the body, and thus they reduced the patient to a state of extreme weakness." See Lind, *An Essay on Diseases Incidental to Europeans in Hot Climates*, 4.

environment—its airs, waters, and places—so humans could survive, if not thrive, in an environment unlike that of their home. "Just like the concept of 'seasoning,' where the first year in the New World was by far the most dangerous," Alan S. Rome observes, "Englishmen needed to be weaned onto their new diet."[58] The process of acclimating to new food began on board ship, where rations held some resemblance to typical English diets—"salt beef, pork, salt fish, butter, cheese, peas, pottage, water gruel, and such kind of victuals, with good biscuits, and six-shilling beer," according to early Virginia immigrant William Wood—but without the more unprocessed local, perishable vegetables and dairy products that would have accompanied such basic fare at home. Wood recommended that travelers also "carry some comfortable refreshing of fresh victual" for their travels, knowing that eventually they would need to become accustomed to the dried and salted foodstuffs imported to Virginia, and the nourishment available there.[59]

Preserving food suitable for the English, and tending to the health of newly arrived countrymen and women, made guarding against the encroachment of Virginia's environment a priority in Jamestown. But, just as the palisades surrounding the Jamestown fort rotted under the influence of the region's water and weather, the boundaries between English bodies and the surrounding land inevitably eroded, making real the threat of the cultural degeneration that Jean Feerick identifies in early modern English colonial accounts.[60] When the English worried whether "those transplanted to distant lands [would] maintain consanguinity with family members in England once their bodies had absorbed the imprint of different climates, diets, and cultures," they were in effect facing the possibility that their class and cultural identity "might be less an inherited essence than a function of place and context."[61]

58 Rome, *The English Embrace of the American Indians*, 104. The illness accompanying seasoning was, in Rome's view, "a superficial adaptation to the climate rather than an important shift in constitution and identity; it was a way of reconciling the influence of the environment with the reluctance to attribute that environment determining power." Similarly, he holds that the adjustment to American-grown crops proved similarly shallow, given that the colonizers insisted on the essential Englishness of their bodies even as their diets changed. See Rome, *The English Embrace of the American Indians*, 108.

59 Michael A. LaCombe, *Political Gastronomy: Food and Authority in the English Atlantic World* (Philadelphia: University of Pennsylvania Press, 2012), 55.

60 Jean Feerick, *Strangers in Blood: Relocating Race in the Renaissance* (Toronto: University of Toronto Press, 2010), 19–20.

61 Feerick, *Strangers in Blood*, 20.

Observing Nature: Seasonal Eating among the Indigenous and English

In this atmosphere, preserving food was a matter of bodily health. As Robert Appelbaum argues, the English food system—even when taking into account feast days and fast days—"was structured to minimize variation and maximize sumptuary regularity" and this "impetus toward regularity was what colonial writers had in mind when they reacted against [Indigenous] customs." The result of this English structure of eating was a system that saw hunger as "an exception, a disruption, a corruption"—which in turn led the English in Virginia to expect "hunger to be as missing from the Americas as it was from Britain."[62] This desire for sameness and predictability in eating in part left the English depending on preserved food—and in the case of Jamestown, imported goods that would need to remain unspoiled through a long overseas voyage—and leads to a failure in the system. "In searching our casked corne, wee found it halfe rotten, and the rest so consumed with the thousand of Rats that ... we knew not how to keepe that little we had," begins one colonist's account that Smith records. "This did drive us all to our wits ende, for there was nothing in the country but what nature afforded."[63] The domestic work of preservation, then, proved key to stabilizing the English body—and indeed, keeping bodies English—in their new environments.

For Wendy Wall, attention to the seasons constituted a central focus of English housewifery, affecting efforts to extend the potential usefulness of fresh ingredients, whether from the field, the store, or the dairy. As a result, Wall argues, "recipes functioned as a site where material and abstract notions of preservation converged," inviting their readers "to manage the physical world through the artful reconfiguration of natural bodies and substances."[64] The result was a cooperative process in which the English housewife worked to modify the impact of time and seasonal weather changes to make foods available when nature would not provide them. This process, moreover, is recorded in recipes that themselves both preserve a record of domestic practices and undergo textual transformation over time. Whether outlining

62 Robert Appelbaum, "Hunger in Early Virginia: Indians and English Facing Off over Excess, Want, and Need," in *Envisioning an English Empire: Jamestown and the Making of the North Atlantic World*, eds. Robert Appelbaum and John Wood Sweet (Philadelphia: University of Pennsylvania Press, 2005), 201, 209, 215. Appelbaum acknowledges that these assumptions about the plentifulness of food obscure questions of labor and economic distribution, and he does not consider how domestic labor plays a role in interrupting the seasonal changes that make food scarce.

63 John Smith, *The Generall Historie of Virginia* (London, 1624), 86.

64 Wall, *Recipes for Thought*, 168.

a technique for making strawberry conserves or for curing a wound, early modern recipes reflect a desire to alter and even stop the changes time brings to physical bodies. And for the English women and men of Jamestown, the concept of saving food and bodies from such decay resonated powerfully.

In Virginia the rhythms of the seasons, not to mention the food practices of local tribes, challenged English notions of food preservation. Settlers like Thomas Hariot and John Smith imagined the Indigenous submitting to the Earth's rhythms rather than attempting to control them by keeping large stores of food for later use. Indeed, their accounts portrayed the Algonquians as passively attuned to the natural cycles of the land, benefitting from the purported "mildnesse of the ayre, the fertilitie of the soyle, and situation of the rivers."[65] Hariot notes the population's willingness to accept what the land had to offer without complaint or greed, describing the tribes near Roanoke as "verye sober in their eatinge, and [drinking], and consequentlye verye longe liued because they doe not oppress nature."[66] For Rachel Winchcombe, Hariot's observation amounts to a suggestion that the Algonquians could prove capable of adopting English ways, since it hints at a respect of the body's humoral balances, even if those are not articulated in their culture.[67] John Smith, on the other hand, observed among the Indigenous a markedly un-English pattern of working with the environment, one that resulted in a direct, distinctly physical impact on Indigenous bodies. He dutifully notes how tribes preserved fish, corn, and berries and outlines modes for planting crops; those activities, however, strike him as less significant than their willingness to accept the changes in food availability—and their own bodies—that came with seasonal cycles. For most of the year, he concludes, "they onely observe times and seasons, and live of what the Country naturally affordeth from hand to mouth."[68] In "observing" nature, Smith imagines the population as conforming to the land, exhibiting an idealized, but extreme and therefore alien, embodiment of Hippocratic notions described in *Airs, Waters, Places.* Oversimplified as they were, these observations depicted Algonquians as making do with what the land provided, seeing no need to worry about what would be available to eat in winter. This view would certainly bring reassurance of plenty to colonizing English ears, even as they sought to impose their own ideas of agriculture on American soil.

65 Smith, *The Generall Historie of Virginia*, 29.

66 Thomas Hariot, "Their sitting at meate," *A Briefe and True Report of the New Found Land of Virginia* (London, 1590), Pl. 16.

67 Rachel Winchcombe, *Encountering Early America* (Manchester: Manchester University Press, 2021), 189–90.

68 Smith, *The Generall Historie of Virginia*, 29.

But Smith struggles to understand the change in physical constitution that comes with "observing" nature's rhythms rather than "keeping" them in a controlled, or at least modified, state. In detailing Indigenous annual activities, Smith notes that, in the summer, "to mend their diet," groups "disperse themselves in small companies, and live upon fish, beasts, crabs, oysters, land Tortoises, strawberries, mulberries, and such like." The movement from one seasonal location to another around the Chesapeake suggests a mobility that contrasted with the permanence Smith and others craved in a Jamestown "plantation," where settlers could remain in a fixed, defensible area customized to fit their needs. Perhaps most surprising, though, is Smith's report of how native bodies change in rhythm with the seasons.

> It is strange to see how their bodies alter with their dyet, even as the deere & wilde beasts they seeme fat and leane, strong and weake. Powhatan their great King, and some others that are provident, rost their fish and flesh upon hurdles as before is expressed, and keepe it till scarce times.[69]

Watching the tribe members as they "observe" nature, Smith notes the fluctuations in their body size from season to season,[70] in direct violation of the English mode of "preserving" the physical, humoral balances fundamental to bodily health. While Smith's final note of "some" of the most "provident" members of the nearest Indigenous tribe drying fish and meat for "scarce times" may serve as a last-minute gesture toward common values and needs, Smith nonetheless marvels at what he sees as the tribes' almost animal-like willingness to accept nature's impact on their bodies, and to see it as a fundamental condition of existence.[71] Rather than preserve food, the Algonquians store it on their bones, preparing themselves for times of hunger through seasonal weight gain that, in William Wood's account, made "their bellies stand forth, ready to split with fullness."[72] Their bodies,

69 Smith, *The Generall Historie of Virginia*, 31. For a valuable reading of Smith's account of these food practices, see Trudy Eden, "Food, Assimilation, and the Malleability of the Human Body in Early Virginia," in *A Centre of Wonders: The Body in Early America,* eds. Janet Moore Lindman and Michele Lise Tarter (Ithaca: Cornell University Press, 2001), 36.

70 Eden, "Food, Assimilation, and the Malleability of the Human Body in Early Virginia," 36.

71 Robert Beverley conveys the Algonquians' different sense of pacing on a smaller time scale, reporting that "They accustom themselves to no set Meals, but eat night and day, when they have plenty of Provisions, or if they have got any thing that is a rarity." Beverley, *The History and Present State of Virginia*, 142; also quoted in Appelbaum, "Hunger in Early Virginia," 196.

72 Wood makes these comments about Algonquian tribes north of Virginia; quoted in Appelbaum, "Hunger in Early Virginia," 196.

that is, illustrate the impact of a different kind of seasoning, showing the effects of environmental change on a more predictable annual scale.

Such accounts suggest a sublimated fear of the impact the Virginia environment could have on English bodies, which the winter of 1609–10 brought to the fore. Though official accounts initially reflected confidence in their food stores, famine and disease descended on the fort in what was quickly labeled the Starving Time. Without other provisions, George Percy recounts in *A Trewe Relacyon*, colonists "fedd uponn horses and other beastes as long as they Lasted" before turning to "vermine as doggs Catts Ratts and myce."[73] For Appelbaum, this suggests a collective slide away from the colony's principled, English eating, illustrating "the regressive behavior of the settlers as they feed themselves first from the valued surpluses, which were to guarantee the condition of alimentary civility they had taken for granted, and then go down the scale and consume less and less edible products, until they are forced to violate the food taboos underlying their nutritional system."[74] Even when forced to "searche the woodes and to feede upon Serpents and snakes and to digge the earthe for wylde and unknowne Rootes," however, the colonists' fare is fresh—newly killed or newly plucked from the earth—rather than preserved, as the most accessible of English foods would be.[75] It is only when the starving turn to shoe leather that they consume preserved flesh of any sort.

Given this progression of consuming what would typically be considered inedible, tales of cannibalism seem inevitable. They are irresistible to historians as well, prompting comparisons to biblical parables and horror stories alike, as well as generating fiery debates about their truthfulness.[76] What matters is that these accounts stuck, resonating both with readers in England and with those seeking to relate the extent of Virginia's suffering. Rachel B.

73 George Percy, "A Trewe Relacyon of the Procedeinges and Occurrentes of Moment which have hapned in Virginia," *Tyler's Quarterly Magazine* 3 (1922): 267, also quoted in LaCombe, *Political Gastronomy*, 52.

74 Appelbaum, "Hunger in Early Virginia," 213, 267.

75 George Percy, "A Trewe Relacyon," 267.

76 LaCombe links the account to biblical stories in LaCombe, *Political Gastronomy*, 53, and Appelbaum reads it as a symbol of absolute extremity—the end not only of the natural means of human subsistence but of the natural restraint on human impulses—in Appelbaum, "Hunger in Early Virginia," 212–14. As Rachel B. Hermann and Gitanjali Shahani note, efforts to assess the veracity of the accounts of cannibalism at the Jamestown fort will never yield definitive answers, though archeological evidence provides evidence of its occurrence. See Rachel B. Hermann, "The 'Tragicall Historie': Cannibalism and Abundance in Colonial Jamestown," *The William and Mary Quarterly* 68, no. 1 (2011): 47–74 and Gitanjali G. Shahani, *Tasting Difference: Food, Race, and Cultural Encounters in Early Modern Literature* (Ithaca: Cornell University Press, 2020).

Hermann sees these stories as allowing the colony's leaders to impress the nature of New World hardships on investors, and to situate those hardships as anomalies rather than everyday[77] (framing them in familiar terms of English famine, as "an exception, a disruption, a corruption," in Appelbaum's words[78]). And indeed, Percy and others readily supply stories of colonists driven by desperation to eat humans, "to doe those things which seame incredible As to digge up dead corpses outt of graves and to eate them and some have Licked upp the Bloode which hathe fallen from their weake fellowes."[79]

But it is the deployment of a recipe, and a recipe for preservation at that, rather than the narrative of cannibalism that is perhaps most surprising in retellings of Jamestown's "disrupting" famine. The most repeated story of cannibalism in the Starving Time involves a settler named Colline who, in Percy's words, "murdered his wyfe Ripped the childe outt of her woambe and threw itt into the River and after chopped the Mother in pieces and salted her for his foode."[80] As Appelbaum points out, Colline remains civilized, even English, in his cannibalism, as gruesome as the story is. He has been "programmed" to "salt" his meat, to put it in storage, and to resign himself to eating it again and again whether he has an appetite for it or not.[81] Colline does not gorge as the Indigenous presumably would; instead, he rations his wife's flesh, preserving it for his future meals as supplies grow even more scarce. John Smith's retelling of the story recognizes the strange civility to the story, playing it for a joke:

> And one amongst the rest did kill his wife, powdered her, and had eaten part of her before it was knowne, for which hee was executed, as hee well deserved; now whether shee was better roasted, boyled or carbonado'd, I know not, but of such a dish as powdered wife I never heard of.[82]

It is not the consumption of human flesh that Smith claims to be shocked by; it is the preservation. Even while the story devalues the woman's life, it expresses a skewed admiration for the domestic skills that might have been among her duties and which, in a switch of gender roles, her husband deployed on her murdered body. While Smith refrains from directly saying he would have cooked the women's flesh over an open flame rather than preserved it in salt,

77 Hermann, "The Tragicall Historie': Cannibalism and Abundance in Colonial Jamestown," 48–49.

78 Appelbaum, "Hunger in Early Virginia," 209.

79 Percy, "A Trewe Relacyon," 267.

80 Percy, "A Trewe Relacyon," 267.

81 Appelbaum, "Hunger in Early Virginia," 214.

82 Smith, *The Generall Historie of Virginia*, 106.

his comments suggest he has his own preferred methods for preparing meats. Smith's story might bring to mind his reports of Algonquian men drying fish over open flames for later consumption, but the modes of preparation he names in his account echo the techniques Jamestown residents would soon read about in Markham's *Countrey Contentments*. Markham offers explicit directions for "ordinary wholsome boild-meats" and for roasting mutton, beef, fish, and poultry, portraying such cooking as everyday in nature;[83] his mention of carbanodos, or meats broiled directly on charcoal, suggest the practice would be less familiar, since it was "first brought out of *Fraunce* as appeares by the name."[84] Smith's incorporation of this domestic knowledge mocks Colline's involvement with homemaking practice while proclaiming his own familiarity with it, all to jokingly suggest that preserving the woman's flesh is a step too far. Powdering her body is unfathomable, Smith implies, because it not just violates moral codes but misapplies usual English household knowledge. Preserving her flesh is excessive, even if it is English.

Smith's report of Colline's act of preservation tries to bring levity to a horrific scene only to raise the specter of fading Englishness among the colonists. The preservative salting signals profound changes, vividly illustrating the unnamed wife's transformation from fertile mother-to-be into preserved food for her husband. The image mocks the notion of rooting English families in the colony, extinguishing life from the woman's body and noting the disposal of her fetus to mark the end of hopes for fertility and growth. Her salted body, however, remains protected, even if temporarily, from decay, subject to the methods of preservation she might have implemented in her own kitchen. Her husband, moreover, is the one who took up the domestic task, and his slippage into kitchenwork further signals Colline's moral and physical decline. The wife's body remains, but her husband's supposedly upstanding English character degrades as he brines her flesh for future consumption.

American Recipe Manuscripts and Dr. Stevens's Water

The power of Dr. Stevens's Water to preserve health must have made it irresistible to those living in a place like the tidewater, where English colonial bodies suffered routine diminishment through sickness and malnourishment, and where the new environment threatened cultural connections to their

83 Markham, *Countrey Contentments, or The English Husvvife*, 47, 53–60.

84 Markham, *Countrey Contentments, or The English Husvvife*, 63.

homeland. Whether this elaborate and powerful cordial water was actually made or used by the earliest English in the region, or simply lingered in the memories of those who read about its preparation, the recipe's promises resonated with Virginia manuscript compilers. Not all recipes that were kept were copied because they were immediately useful, as we have seen; they could instead signal a connection to the past, or an impulse to prepare for events in the future, or simply hold narrative appeal. Any of these reasons could have led the keeper of *A Booke of Sweetmeats* to dutifully copy out directions for making Dr. Stevens's Water, echoing Markham's phrasing in a way that suggests *Countrey Contentments* as the recipe's source. The Virginia-based collection, bound with a second manuscript principally in the same hand entitled *A Booke of Cookery*, has long been associated with Martha Washington, though Karen Hess has traced the manuscript to much earlier American roots. She associates the compilation with Frances Culpeper, also known as Lady Berkeley, which situates the collection in Virginia during the 1650s, if not before.[85] Eventually, through marriage, the book made its way to First Lady Martha Parke Custis Washington, who took ownership of it with her first marriage in 1749, then brought it to the home of her second husband, George Washington, before giving it to her granddaughter, Nellie Curtis, in 1799.[86]

While a relationship between the Dr. Stevens's Waters found in the Berkeley/Washington collection and Markham's book is impossible to prove beyond a doubt, the documented availability of *Countrey Contentments* in the colony makes the book a likely candidate as a source for the manuscript's version of the recipe. Hess sees parallels between the Berkeley/Washington manuscript's version, and the one appearing in Cogan's 1584 *Haven of Health*,[87] and indeed such a relationship would account of the manuscripts' omission of Markham's oregano. Either version's story of the cordial's power to extend life beyond the short number of years typical for colonists would have been a tale too enticing to ignore. But the manuscript's echoing of Markham's distinctive verb *bray*, along with the documented presence of *Countrey Contentments* on the continent, suggests that this Virginian text echoes his version.[88]

85 Hess, *Martha Washington's Booke of Cookery*, 460–62.

86 Hess, *Martha Washington's Booke of Cookery*, 3. The manuscript is housed in the Historical Society of Pennsylvania, in the collection entitled *Historical Society of Pennsylvania Collection of George Washington Family Papers*.

87 Hess, *Martha Washington's Booke of Cookery*, 404, where she also notes the appearances of Dr. Stevens's Water in other early modern printed books.

88 Similarly, Cogan appends a recommendation to the recipe, suggesting that using half the herbs and twice the spices yields better results, and that "Sacke or very strong Ale" is a better base than wine. See Cogan, *The Hauen of Health*, 232.

To make Doctor Steuens water.	To Make Doctor Steephens his Cordiall Water
To make that soueraine water which was first inuented by Doctor *Steuens*, in the same forme as he deliuered the Receite to the Arch-bishop of *Canturbury*, a little before the death of the said Doctor. Take a gallon of good Gaskoine wine, then take Ginger, Galuingale, Synamon, Nutmegges, Graines, Cloues bruised, Fennell seede, Carrawaie seede, Origanum; of euery of them a like quantitie, that is to say a dramme: then take Sage, wild Margerum, Peny-royall, Mints, Red-roses, Time, Pellitory, Rosemary, wild-time, Cammomill, Lauender, of each of them one handfull: then braie the spices small, and bruise the hearbes and put all into the wine, and let it stand so 12 houres, only stirre it diuers times, then distill it by a Limbecke, and keepe the first water by it selfe for that is the best, then keepe the second water for that is good, and for the last neglect it not, for it is very wholsom though the worst of the three. Now for the vertue of this water it is this, it comforteth the spirits and vitall parts, and helpeth all inward diseases that commeth of colde, it is good against the shaking of the palsey, and cureth the contraction of sinnewes, and helpeth the conception of women that be barraine; it killeth the wormes within the body, it cureth the cold cough, it helpeth the tooth-ache, it comforteth the stomacke and cureth the old dropsie; it helpeth the stone in the bladder and in the reines, it helpeth a stinking breath: and whosoeuer vseth this water moderately and not too often, preserueth him in good liking, and will make him seeme young in olde age. With this water Doctor *Steuens* preserued his owne life vntill such extreame age, that he could neither goe nor ride, and he continued his life being bed-rid fiue yeeres, when other Physicions did iudge hee could not liue one yeere, which he did confesse a little before his death; saying: that if he were sicke at anie time, he neuer vsed any thing but this water only; and also the Archbishop of *Canterbury* vsed it, and found such goodnesse in it that he liued till he was not able to drink of a cup, but sucked his drink through a hollow pipe of siluer. This water will be much the better if it be set in the sunne all summer.	Take a gallon of the best gascoyne wine; then take cloves, ginger, gallinggall, cinnamon, & nutmeggs, graynes, anny seeds, fennell seeds, carraway seeds, of each a dram. then take wild time, lavender, sage, mints, hysope, red roses, garden time, pellitory of the wall, & rosemary, of each one handfull. bray the hearbs small, & stamp the spices alltogether very small & put all into your wine & cover it close for 12 hours, except when you stir it, which must be often. distill it in A limbeck, & keep the first water by it selfe, it beeing the strongest. but of the second sort, you may drink A greater quantety. The Vertues of this Water This water comforts the vitall spirits, it perserveth the Joynts, & helpeth inward disseases comeing of cold, it is good against the shaking of the palsie, it cureth the contraction of the sinews, it helpeth conception in women that are barren, it killeth worms in the body, it comforteth the stomack, it is good for the cold dropsie & stone in the bladder & in the reynes, it helpeth a stinking breath. and whosever useth this water sometimes, but not too often, it preserveth theyr health & causeth them to look young.
–Markham, *Countrey Contentments or The English Husvvife*[89]	–*A Booke of Sweetmeats*, Berkeley/Washington manuscript[90]

89 Markham, *Countrey Contentments or The English Husvvife*, 29–30.

90 As transcribed in Hess, *Martha Washington's Booke of Cookery*, 402–4. I have, however, expanded common abbreviations.

At its most basic, Dr. Stevens's Water depends on preservation—of the distillation of herbs and spices in wine—for its powers. As Wendy Wall has shown, distillation was conceptualized as a mode of reducing ingredients to their most powerful essences, delaying their decay in the process.[91] Extending the ingredients'—and patient's—liveliness takes time, though, since the recipe asks for the herbs and spices to steep twelve hours before going through three separate rounds of distillation. Versions of the recipe that suggest the water be left in the sun for an even longer period—in Markham's case, "all summer"—require an even greater investment of the maker's time. This patience pays off, or so the recipe promises, by enabling the maker to extend the lives of those around her, even if these people survive without the power to move in their own rights. Their bodies continue to foster life; even when terribly impaired, the bedridden Dr. Stevens and Archbishop remain proud of their medically induced endurance among the living.

Dr. Stevens's Water earned its place among the conserves and pickles that populate many Virginia's manuscript cookbooks, preserving the strength of English bodies surrounded by airs, waters, and places they were only slowly learning to tolerate. Once included in these manuscripts, moreover, the cordial became an entrenched feature in early American compilations, though its ingredients varied in some recountings. Curiously, no version suggests using the water to treat suffering during the seasoning process, though many versions declare effectiveness against symptoms linked to the condition. The version in a manuscript dated ca. 1700, and associated with the recipe-keeping Randolph family of Virginia, contains a "Doca. Stevens Water" that follows Cogan's advice in the printed 1584 *Haven of Health*, using sack as its base and folding North American sassafras into a modified list of two dozen herbs. A 1744 manuscript, also possibly linked to the Randolphs, adheres more closely to the Berkeley/Washington version, using the more well-established list of herbs but suggesting using equal parts brandy and "Gasking wine."[92]

91 See Wendy Wall, "Distillation: Transformations in and out of the Kitchen," in *Renaissance Food from Rabelais to Shakespeare: Culinary Readings and Culinary Histories*, ed. Joan Fitzpatrick (Burlington: Ashgate, 2010), 89–104.

92 The two Virginia manuscript versions of the recipe are transcribed in Harbury, *Colonial Virginia's Cooking Dynasty*, 220. See the manuscript *Cookbook*, ca. 1700, Virginia Museum of History & Culture at the Virginia Historical Society MS 5:5 Un 3:4, Virginia Historical Society, Richmond, VA; I am grateful to Matthew Guillen, Reference Coordinator for providing a copy of the recipe "To Make Doca. Stevens Watter" from this collection, whose pages are not numbered. The 1744 manuscript is cataloged as *Manuscript Cookbook*, eighteenth-century MESDA MS VA.M MFm 5A at the Museum of Early Southern Decorative Arts (MESDA) Research Center, Old Salem Museums and Gardens, Winston-Salem, NC; I am also grateful for Kim Wilson May for providing me with images of that manuscript's "Doctor Stephens's Water" from page 44. Both

The colonial manuscripts, however, omit any lengthy discussion of the water's virtues; most striking, they make no mention of the water's preservative power. Not only is the Archbishop of Canterbury gone, so is Dr. Stevens himself. The recipe endures, but it no longer asks users to imagine its near-magical ability to help patients survive to an extremely advanced age. The recipe may itself be preserved, but its powers have faded away in these later editions, suggesting that the local users of Virginia had seen no evidence of its elaborate claims. The possibility of lingering bedridden may also have simply lost its appeal to North American users, whose omission of such claims also sever a connection to the Archbishop of Canterbury. For these new manuscript compilers, omitting the stories once linked to Dr. Stevens's Water preserves what is valuable about the medicine, even as it loosens ties to the English culture that produced it.

Preserving Life the Algonquian Way

Despite the link between Englishness and Dr. Stevens's Water, the recipe's fantasy of extreme bodily preservation is not unique in the New World. In fact, George Percy perpetuates the tale of an elder of the Pamunkey tribe who outlasts even Dr. Stevens. Though his account does not gain the same resonance as the cordial water recipe—which creates a preserving distillation which lingers in manuscripts and print, perhaps beyond its usefulness—Percy's account describes a far more active elder, one who lived beyond 160 years. This makes him not only older than Dr. Stevens in even the most extreme retellings, but older than the recipe for his water would have likely been at the time. Percy tells us, in charged but admiring language:

> The Savages beare their yeeres well, for when wee were at Pamonkies, wee saw a Savage by their report was above eight score yeeres of age. His eyes were sunke into his head, having never a tooth in his mouth, his haire all gray with a reasonable bigge beard, which was as white as any snow. It is a Miracle to see a Savage have any haire on their faces, I never saw, read, nor heard, any have the like before. This savage was as lustie and went as fast as any of us, which was strange to behold.[93]

manuscripts are associated with ancestors of Mary Randolph, author of the 1824 cookbook *The Virginia Housewife*, which has recipes for preserves, pickles, and cordial waters but contains no mention of Dr. Stevens's Water. See Randolph, *The Virginia Housewife*.

93 George Percy, "Observations by Master George Percy, 1607," in *Narratives of Early Virginia, 1606–1625*, ed. Lyon Gardiner Tyler (New York: Scribner's, 1907), 19.

This man is no Dr. Stevens, for he is "lustie" rather than bedridden and able to keep pace with Englishmen no more than a third of his age. Among the characteristics most striking to Percy, though, is the man's facial hair—something that he associates more with Europeans like himself than the Indigenous in America. The Pamunkey man does not resemble his own kin so much as he does an elderly Englishman, with white hair and a beard, yet his endurance surpasses anything that Percy might expect of his own countrymen.

Percy's anecdote suggests an aura of endurance around this Pamunkey man that no English person could match. And while he makes no such claims for the Algonquian population as a whole, his story suggests a realization that, in the long run, the English are at a disadvantage in Virginia. The Virginia atmosphere, after all, definitely took its toll, on the English as well as on the items they brought with them. The fate of the women on the 1620 and 1621 ships is instructive. Alice Burges and Ann Tanner disappear from records after disembarking at Jamestown. Perhaps even more striking is the vanishing of Elizabeth Markham, a sixteen-year-old woman purported to be the daughter of Gervase Markham, who arrived at the plantation in 1621, a year after her father's books landed in the colony.[94] She disappears upon reaching Virginia, never heard from again after setting foot on American soil. While this could be a sign of her success as a Jamestown bride—of a name changed in marriage, and a fruitful life in the years that followed in a new home—her English identity nonetheless vanishes, along with any distinct connection to the foundational, influential domestic texts that bore her father's name. No traces remain of her presence among the English colonists, and no evidence remains of her perpetuating the household practices upon which her father's notoriety rested. She does not even enjoy the infamous end associated with Colline's preserved wife. Like so many other occupants of the Virginia tidewater, Elizabeth Markham evades any documentation—not even in the form of court records or known domestic recipes—that would have perpetuated, if not preserved, her story. Her father's texts, meanwhile, linger, much like Dr. Stevens.

Despite its complexity, the recipe for Dr. Stevens's Water endured in America, suggesting that settlers valued its emphasis on the English body's potential to live to old age even if they refrained from recording extreme stories of the cure's potency. Such efforts to preserve this and other imported

94 See Martha McCartney, *Documentary History of Jamestown Island*, Jamestown Archaeological Assessment, 1992–96, National Park Service (Williamsburg, VA: Colonial Williamsburg Foundation, 2000), 3:63, 233, 357.

recipes illustrate a determination to maintain the Englishness of settler bodies, even in surroundings different from the ones that were best suited for their health, at least according to the humoral theories of *Airs, Waters, Places*. In doing so, manuscript recipes called upon home preserving practices and cordials like Dr. Stevens's miraculous water to underscore a connection to England that no doubt faded with every year in America. Clinging to these recipes and their depiction of English survival, and even longevity, the people who preserved such English recipes in America resisted entanglement with their environment, instead imagining themselves as intertwined with their forerunners across the sea. Markham's recipe for Dr. Stevens's Water—like many versions of the cordial—situated the cure in the English landscape of the Virginia housewives' birthplaces, or, for later settler generations, in the ancestral homes of their foremothers. Copying the recipe into their collections, these Virginia women insisted on a physical connection between their bodies and their English roots, resisting the pull of their lived environment in hopes of imposing their ancestral narratives upon the surrounding tidewater.

5. Traveling Diseases, Imported Cures: Rheumatism and Sassafras in Home Medical Manuscripts

Abstract: This chapter examines the role of sassafras in keeping English colonies in America thriving. In America, sassafras helped settlers survive scurvy and the process of seasoning. The Virginia Company's efforts to raise the reputation of sassafras as a cure succeeded not just in increasing the plant's appearance in medical recipes in manuscripts; it also increased the appearance of diseases for the plant to cure. As recipes requiring sassafras became common in manuscript collections, that is, so did the appearance of conditions identified as "rheumatism" that the plant excelled in curing. The Frankland family's collection characterized rheumatism as an American disease and used sassafras to cure it, reinforcing notions that the places that fostered illnesses provided the best cures for those diseases.

Keywords: University of Pennsylvania Ms. Codex 644; Frankland family; scurvy; Nicolás Monardes; Indigenous knowledge; newspapers

During their attempts to establish themselves in North America, English colonies relied on narratives of health not just to convince potential settlers to take up residence, but to create markets for the materials gathered and produced there. Financial success depended on harvesting and selling resources, often botanical, obtained from these new outposts. Trade with Indigenous people could bring access to goods already perceived as valuable in European ports, and it could also supply plants to answer needs that English customers did not yet know they had. The environmental and cultural markers that rendered a plant's place of origin distinct and meaningful to Indigenous people were gradually stripped away in this process, even though it was the place of origin that initially made these American materials

Nunn, Hillary M. *Recipes on the Move in Early Modern England and British North America: Domestic Medicine, Mobility, and Manuscript Culture*. Amsterdam: Amsterdam University Press, 2025.
DOI 10.5117/9789463723398_CH05

desirable in Europe. As Daniela Bleichmar explains, "Products were carried from the New World to Europe, and at times some information regarding their use traveled with them, but the web of beliefs and associations that made these objects meaningful to Amerindian societies were left behind."[1] As valuable as medical materials from the Americas proved in Europe, that value depended on perceptions of usefulness for curing diseases known on the eastern side of the Atlantic. This applied even when the diseases themselves were thought to be imports. As Edith Snook points out, however, the reigning belief that God provided cures through the landscape erases Indigenous peoples—specifically Indigenous women—from "the creation, possession, and communication of medical knowledge."[2] Rather than credit Indigenous learning and tradition, accounts of New World cures worked to explain their effectiveness in relation to long-held European knowledge frameworks.[3]

The incorporation of sassafras into English medical practices illustrates this process of absorbing Indigenous knowledge, which survived translation even when the names of those who communicated its value did not. As Clare Griffin argues, the establishment of sassafras as a part of European health discourse ran parallel to the construction of the Americas in the colonizers' imagination. When the Spanish arrived in Florida, they learned from French explorers of a tree that neither European group had encountered before, which the French labeled *sassafras* even though the Timucua, who taught them the plant's uses, called it *pauame*. The Spanish followed the French example, and their accounts spread sassafras's reputation as an antifebrile drug. The name *sassafras* stuck for Europeans, even when they learned more about the plant's uses from the Tacaacuru of Georgia, who called it *wissoe*, and the Powhatans near Jamestown, who called it *winauk*. Gerard's *Herball* omits those names, but notes that the Spanish and the French used the word *sassafras* for the plant that "Indians in their tongue" called "*Pauame*."[4] As Europeans were taking "*wissoe*, *winauk*, and *pauame*,

1 Daniela Bleichmar, "Books, Bodies, and Fields: Sixteenth-Century Transatlantic Encounters with New World *Materia Medica*," in *Colonial Botany: Science, Commerce, and Politics*, eds. Londa Schiebinger and Claudia Swan (Philadelphia: University of Pennsylvania Press, 2005), 98.

2 See Snook's valuable examination of Lady Grace Mildmay's use of guaiacum, in Edith Snook, "Grace Mildmay's Recipes and Indigenous Knowledge in the Early Modern Atlantic World," *Atlantic Studies* 19, no. 2 (2022): 225.

3 For discussion of the impact of translation in the movement of medical cures, see Rankin's study regarding works by Monardes, in Alisha Rankin, "New World Drugs and the Archive of Practice: Translating Nicolás Monardes in Early Modern Europe," *Osiris* 37 (2022): 68–88; also see Pablo F. Gómez, "[Un]Muffled Histories: Translating Bodily Practices in the Early Modern Caribbean," *Osiris* 37 (2022): 233–50.

4 John Gerard, *The Herball or Generall History of Plantes* (London, 1633), 1525.

and making them into sassafras," Griffin explains, "they were similarly creating the New World" from "a combination of their experiences in the real world of the early modern Americas and their preconceptions."[5] And, when Gerard notes that he based his illustration of the plant on a "branch taken from a little tree, which grew in the Garden of Master *Wilmote* at Bow," he makes clear that material traces of those encounters could develop a life of their own once transported to England.[6]

The results of this appropriation appear in recipe manuscripts kept in English settler homes in the Americas as early as the seventeenth century. While these collections reflect local use, the cures they preserve can also be traced traveling *away* from North America, accompanying their owners as business and kinship obligations compelled them—and later their American born children—to England. Medical ingredients and healthcare knowledge traveled together across the Atlantic, and this traffic flowed in both directions. But even when a recipe manuscript's journeys can be mapped—as is the case with the Frankland family manuscript, examined in this chapter—there is rarely much certainty as to when particular recipes made their way into these collections. Because they were often compiled over decades, if not generations, the location a recipe keeper might have occupied while writing a cure into her book is difficult, if not impossible, to determine, even when the medicine might call for ingredients associated with specific environments. As we have seen, one recipe on a manuscript page can omit all obvious clues to place, only to be followed by one that seems to reference multiple different locales.[7] Many seventeenth-century English-language recipes mix ingredients imported from American colonies with materials long considered staples of English healthcare, resulting in cures with a new, distinctly American tinge.

In England, the increased presence of American ingredients in recipe manuscripts signals a key shift in perceptions of a local environment's connections to illness, and its cures. The incorporation of these imported materials highlights a new elasticity in the perceived links connecting bodies, diseases, and the places that shaped them. Colonialism, after all, reinforced awareness that disease could travel from one place to another despite the long-held notions that particular ecosystems could cause specific ailments; the trade routes that developed during the period depended on

5 Clare Griffin, "Disentangling Commodity Histories: Pauame and Sassafras in the Early Modern Global World," *Journal of Global History* 15, no. 1 (2020): 1–3.

6 Gerard, *The Herball or Generall History of Plantes*, 1524.

7 See chapter 2.

the notion that botanical cures could travel as well, and that uses could be found for those plants upon arrival. Manuscript recipe books linked to households in England offer a valuable glimpse into the welcome these traveling botanical ingredients received, revealing the healthcare uses that people residing in London and the surrounding countryside found for materials imported from the Americas.

Illnesses and afflictions, moreover, proved just as mobile as the treatments that could cure them. Such was the case with the condition labeled rheumatism, whose definition and treatment evolved in the English imagination as more cures were found for it among American plants. As the connections between rheumatism and its New World treatments solidified in English thinking, the illness itself became increasingly associated with the American colonies. Rheumatism and sassafras made their way into English medical discourse together in the seventeenth and eighteenth centuries, suggesting that the arrival of sassafras in England coincided with a rising visibility, and even a new definition, of the disease—a disease that the plant could, conveniently, help to treat. The symptoms newly attached to rheumatism linked the condition to the North American continent and the damp, cold environments thought prevalent there. The bark of the American sassafras tree becomes a key to treating this brand of redefined, lingering rheumatism, which transformed from a mild congestive complaint long familiar in England into a chronic condition incorporating the swelling, joint pain, and tooth loss of scurvy, another disease that English people linked with faraway places. Scurvy, the archetypical disease of ocean crossings, was itself often treated with concoctions containing sassafras, and it shared increasing space with rheumatism in English recipe manuscripts during the age of colonization. The increasing use of the term *rheumatism*, and the arrival of American ingredients in England, suggest a correspondence between colonial activities and the disease, one that itself was often defined as a wandering pain that left sufferers uncomfortable in their own skins.

Rheumatism in the Frankland Manuscript

No recipe collection more clearly illustrates American botanical ingredients' place at the juncture of the mutating perceptions of rheumatism and the changing world of trade than Lady Frankland's eighteenth-century recipe manuscript. Begun approximately a century after the founding of Jamestown, this collection provides a glimpse of how recipes traveled not only to the

Americas and within the colonies, but out of the Americas as well.[8] The manuscript underscores the lasting perception of biological and cultural connection between people in England and white settlers in North America, since its recipes were imagined as effective for both groups. The inside of the Frankland manuscript's front cover bears an inscription identifying it as "Grandmama Lady Frankland's Receipt Book," leading Marissa Nicosia to connect the collection to Lady Sarah Frankland, born Sarah Rhett in Charleston, South Carolina around 1724. The Rhetts were long established in the colony, operating sugar and rice plantations that depended on the labor of enslaved workers. In 1743, in Charleston, Sarah married Sir Thomas Frankland, fifth baronet (1718–84); he had been born in the East Indies but retained close enough ties with his ancestral home in Yorkshire to represent Thirsk in Parliament later in life. In fact, Sarah was living in England in 1750, seven years after she married, at the time of her first son's birth; she died there in 1808. Where she lived when she began recording her recipes is unclear, and, given that she and her descendants added to her book in later years, declaring the collection either American or English in origin would be an oversimplification. Frankland's recipe collection instead traces the impact of her travels and of the journeys her husband undertook, as well as the evolving traditions of her birthplace. The text incorporates American ingredients as well as East Indian curries and rice dishes informed by African influences, serving, in Nicosia's words, "as a contact zone between Britain, the Americas, Africa, and the East Indies."[9] The recipe collection, moreover, continued to travel after her death, eventually landing back in the Americas, at the Kislak Center at the University of Pennsylvania. By curious chance, Sarah's manuscript also perpetuates the traditions of family recipe keeping in another way; her husband's great grandmother, Arabella Belasyse Frankland, was sister to Grace Belasyse, whose recipe collection is discussed in chapter 2.[10]

The Frankland medical recipes incorporate many ingredients associated with transatlantic trade, such as Peruvian bark, tobacco, and Virginia

8 Lady Frankland, *Recipe Book*, 1750–1825, University of Pennsylvania Ms. Codex 644, University of Pennsylvania, Philadelphia, PA.

9 Marisa Nicosia, "Slaveholding, Seasoning, and the Circulation of Culinary Knowledge in the Frankland Family Receipt Book," in *American Contact: Objects of Intercultural Encounters and the Boundaries of Book History*, eds. Rhae Lynn Barnes and Glenda Goodman (Philadelphia: University of Pennsylvania Press, 2023), 142–50, esp. 144.

10 Thomas Frankland, fifth baronet, was son of Sir Henry Frankland (1690–1728), who was son of Thomas Frankland, 2nd baronet (1665–1726), whose mother was Arabella Belasyse Frankland (ca. 1640–87), sister of Grace Belasyse Saunderson, Lady Castleton (ca. 1635–67). The two women grew up together at Newburgh Priory.

snakeroot in a cure for the ague,[11] but the sassafras tea involved in a treatment for rheumatism offers especially vivid proof of the new portability of both cures and disease. The rheumatism cure is labeled explicitly as "American," suggesting an intact biological commonality between people in England and the colonists who journeyed there to establish transatlantic outposts. Appearing on the manuscript's later pages, the rheumatism recipe may have been added years after the book's start, and likely in England after Sarah's move there. The very fact that the Franklands included the recipe at all indicates that they expected it would likely prove effective when it traveled to new locales to treat different people. The recipe's "American" title establishes a distinct point of origin while implying that other recipes in the collection are *not* American:

> A famous American Receipt for the
> Rheumatism. £100 has been given for this receipt
>
> Take of Garlic two cloves of Gum ammoniac
> one drachm. Blend them by bruising together
> make them into three boluses with
> fair water & swallow them, one at night
> & one in the morning. drink while taking
> this recipt Sassafras Tea made very
> strong so as to have the Tea pot filled
> with chips – This is generally found to
> banish the Rhumatism, & even contractions
> in the joints, in a very few times taking[12]

Even if recorded while in South Carolina, the "American Receipt for the Rheumatism" stands out, associated with a different environment than the collection's other cures. If recorded in England, the rheumatism recipe openly declares itself an import, one uprooted from its American home and brought to Lady Frankland's attention—just as one of its key ingredients, sassafras, would have been. And, just like sassafras, the recipe itself is a product of trade. It is labeled as a purchase—someone, if not Lady Frankland, supposedly paid the dear price of £100 for rather straightforward instructions to combine gum and garlic into small balls, or boluses, to eat while drinking sassafras tea.

11 Frankland, *Recipe Book*, 1750–1825, University of Pennsylvania Ms. Codex 644, 37r.

12 Frankland, *Recipe Book*, 1750–1825, University of Pennsylvania Ms. Codex 644, 36r.

In naming an entire hemisphere as its origin, the "American Receipt for the Rheumatism" claims authority from transatlantic trade even as it calls out the expense of imported medical knowledge. While buying medical recipes was certainly not unusual—patients and caregivers, after all, routinely paid apothecaries for their recipe-making expertise, and customers commonly bought printed books that contained recipes for treatments—the specifics of this exchange sets this American receipt apart. Its claim to monetary value, reminiscent of modern urban legends of exorbitant prices for luxury department store cookie recipes, links the cure directly to commerce, rather than to the neighborly or familial exchange of knowledge often seen in manuscript recipe collections. No individual name—whether of a family member, local doctor, or Indigenous trading partner—is attached to the recipe, leaving its "American" source less precisely identified than many attributions in manuscript collections. The recipe declares itself a product, something to be bought and sold just like the ingredients it contains. The inclusion of the "American Receipt for the Rheumatism" in a manuscript betrays an evident delight in evading market forces, slyly saving its readers a substantial amount of money.[13] For the manuscript's reader, the recipe presents itself as a kind of bargain, a circumvention of the marketplace—the revelation, presumably without the cost—of valuable knowledge, something that looks like a trade secret.

Rather than name an individual as the source of its knowledge, this rheumatism cure relies on its association with a colonized place of origin, and generic "fame," for its credibility. This is even more remarkable given that only one of its three ingredients can easily claim American roots. While sassafras is closely linked to North American trade, the recipe's other ingredients hail from the eastern side of the Atlantic. Garlic was likely to be locally grown or even found in English fields,[14] while the fact that gum ammoniac, a sticky resin extracted from a plant native to North Africa,[15]

13 Commenting on the Nieman Marcus Cookie recipe rumor, which features a customer unknowingly paying $250 for a recipe she then spreads for free, Fine and Turner argue that "Part of the story's appeal comes from the willingness of the abused consumer to turn the tables on the big corporation. When we pass the recipe along, we participate in the customer's revenge." See Gary Alan Fine and Patricia A. Turner, *Whispers on the Color Line: Rumor and Race in America* (Berkeley: University of California Press, 2001), 11.

14 As Gerard notes, garlic is "planted in gardens of the small cloves in November and December" and wild varieties grow in England like Crow Garlick and Mountain Garlick. See Gerard, *The Herball or Generall History of Plantes*, 177. He does, however, offer descriptions of garlic species found in other parts of the world. See Gerard, *The Herball or Generall History of Plantes*, 179–82.

15 Le Fèbure states that African gum ammoniac is "taken from a feculaceous plant growing in that part of *Africa* where formerly was the Temple of *Jupiter Ammon*, whence it had also the name";

owes its presence in England to more established routes of trade is completely overlooked in the recipe's title. This focus on the recipe's American origins further emphasizes both sassafras and the knowledge of its use are imports proving key to its effectiveness. The link is no accident either, as suggested by the recipe's second appearance in the Frankland manuscript. Turn the page twice, and the recipe appears again, in the same handwriting, without reference to price but with its American origins front and center:

> American Receipt for the Rheumatism &
> Contraction of the joints –
>
> 2 cloves of Garlic – 1 drachm of gum ammoniac –
> Bruise them together in a mortar – make the mixture into
> 2 or 3 bolusses with spring water. Take one every night &
> & morning – and drink while regularly taking these bolusses, very
> Strong sassafras tea.[16]

The second appearance of the cure in Frankland's manuscript is notable but not unique. Repetition of cures occurs, as we have seen in the Castleton text.[17] But what is notable is the place of the second version of the sassafras-based

see Nicaise Le Fèbure, *A Compendious Body of Chymistry* (London, 1662), 77. Also see Nancy Cox and Karin Dannehl, *Dictionary of Traded Goods and Commodities 1550–1820* (Wolverhampton: University of Wolverhampton, 2007), accessed September 17, 2019. The *OED* asserts that first appearance of the term "gum ammoniac" is in directions to combine the resin with garlic to make watercolor paint, citing Peacham's use in 1627, but it appears in the earlier printing of Peacham's work; see Henry Peacham, *The Gentlemans Exercise* (London, 1612), 71. More general references to *ammoniac* appear even earlier, as far back as 1420. See definitions A.2. and B.1 of *ammoniac*, "ammoniac, adj. and n.," in *Oxford English Dictionary*, accessed June 18, 2022.

16 Frankland, *Recipe Book*, 1750–1825, University of Pennsylvania Ms. Codes 644, 37v. Versions of this recipe appear in at least three other manuscripts, both dated later and compiled in England. The first is in *Book of Receipts*, 1731, Virginia Tech Ms 2008-024, Virginia Tech University, Blacksburg, VA, 35; if this date is correct, this manuscript would have the earliest version of this recipe, but there are several hand changes before the rheumatism recipe's appearance. It is titled "the famous American Receipt for the Rheumatism" which ends by repeating "it is very famous in [A]merica" and notes the cost. The Szathmary Culinary Manuscripts and Cookbooks collection includes a manuscript, dated in the 1800s, with a version of the recipe entitled "An American receipt for Rheumatism, which very seldom fails" which does not include a price. See *English Household and Medicinal Book*, 1800s, University of Iowa, Iowa City, IA, 7. The recipe, without price, also occurs in *A Receipt Book of Mrs. Johnson, 1741/2*, 99v. The collection, which migrated at some point to Canada, likely came to include the rheumatism recipe in the late eighteenth century. See Nathalie Cooke and Kathryn Harvey, eds., *The Johnson Family Treasury: A Collection of Household Recipes and Remedies, 1741–1848* (Oakville, ON: Rock's Mills Press, 2015), 178.

17 See chapter 2.

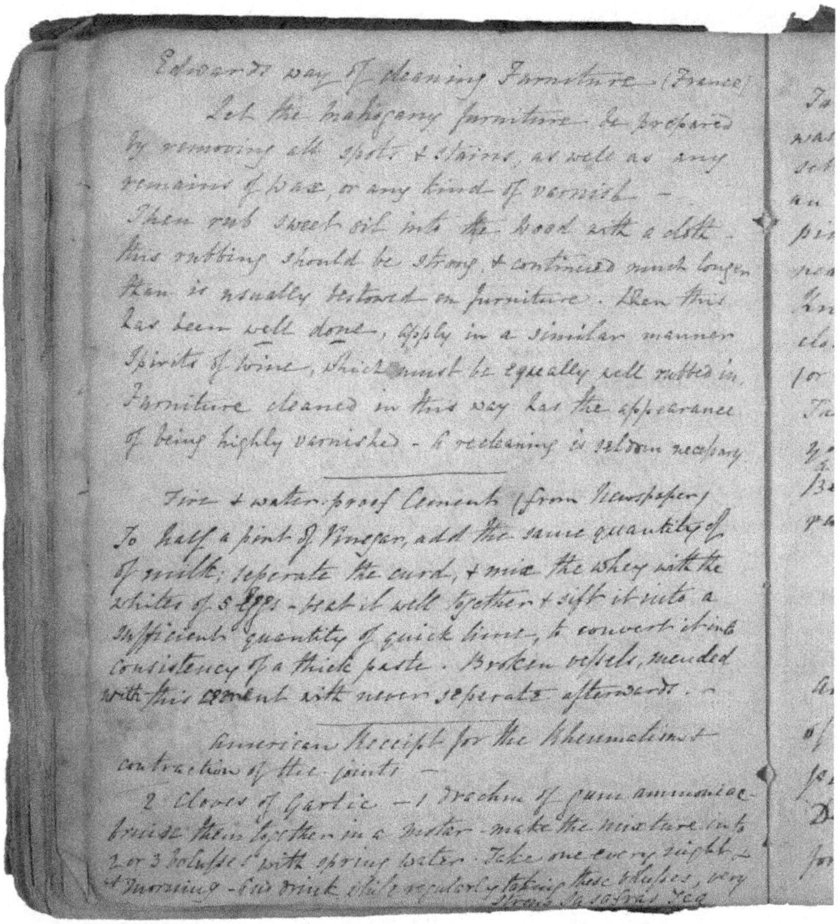
Edwards way of cleaning Furniture (France)
Let the mahogany furniture be prepared
by removing all spots + stains, as well as any
remains of wax, or any kind of varnish –
Then rub sweet oil into the wood with a cloth.
this rubbing should be strong, + continued much longer
than is usually bestowed on furniture. When this
has been well done, apply in a similar manner
Spirits of wine, which must be equally well rubbed in.
Furniture cleaned in this way has the appearance
of being highly varnished – a recleaning is seldom necessary

Fire + water proof Cement (from Newspaper)
To half a pint of Vinegar, add the same quantity of
of milk; seperate the curd, + mix the whey with the
whites of 5 Eggs – beat it well together + sift it into a
sufficient quantity of quick lime, to convert it into
consistency of a thick paste. Broken vessels, mended
with this cement will never seperate afterwards. –

American Receipt for the Rheumatism +
contraction of the joints –
2 Cloves of Garlic – 1 drachm of gum ammoniac
bruise them together in a mortar – make the mixture into
2 or 3 bolusses with spring water. Take one every night
+ morning – & to drink while regularly taking these bolusses, very
strong Sassafras Tea

Figure 4. The second appearance of "American Receipt for the Rheumatism" in the Frankland manuscript, just below "Fire and water proof Cement (from Newspaper)." Lady Frankland, *Recipe Book*, 1750–1825, University of Pennsylvania Ms. Codex 644, University of Pennsylvania, Philadelphia, 37v. Courtesy of the Kislak Center at the University of Pennsylvania.

recipe. Directly above the second rheumatism recipe appear instructions for making "Fire and water proof Cement (from Newspaper)" (figure 4). The manuscript's owner presumably copied this recipe from a print source, raising the possibility that neighboring recipes came from similar circulated materials as well.

And indeed, further investigation shows that "The Famous American Receipt for the Rheumatism" appears in several London newspapers, published all on the same date—June 1, 1766, a day when Lady Frankland would have been living in England. *The London Magazine*, *The Gentleman's Magazine*, *The Royal Magazine*, and *The Universal Magazine* ran largely identical versions of the cure, with the same ingredients and procedures but without the hundred-pound price in the headline. With the exception of spelling, the body of first version in the Frankland manuscript adheres to the newspapers' presentation almost word for word, omitting only the print versions' option to make "two or three" boluses and settling on three. Each printed version, moreover, ends with the claim that "It is very famous in *America*, and an hundred pounds have been given for the receipt."[18] Such copying of print recipes into manuscript is not unusual, as the presence of Dr. Stevens's Water illustrates in the previous chapter, and collecting from newspapers proved popular for manuscript recipe compilers in the eighteenth century.[19] The appearance in a London print forum could even help explain the recipe's title, since incorporation of "American" might have made the cure seem more innovative and desirable, though none of the newspapers situate the recipes in a particularly attention-getting spot.

The multiple appearances of this remedy make clear that recipes crossed oceans in both directions, and in fact this cure managed to zigzag across the Atlantic several times during Frankland's lifetime. In 1768—shortly after those four London instances of "The Famous American Receipt for the Rheumatism" printed in 1766—the recipe appears in *Poor Richard Improved*, an almanac published under the pseudonym Richard Saunders and long associated with Benjamin Franklin, who happened to be in London in 1766.[20]

18 "The Famous American Receipt for the Rheumatism," *London Magazine: or, Gentleman's Monthly Intelligencer* (June 1, 1766): 324. The text is identical in "The Famous American Receipt for the Rheumatism," and *The Universal Magazine of Knowledge and Pleasure* (June 1, 1766): 329, and nearly so in "The Famous American Receipt for the Rheumatism," *Royal Magazine* (June 1, 1766): 300. *The Gentleman's Magazine* contains the same recipe, but uses numerals to quote the price at "100*l*. for this Receipt"; see "The Famous American Receipt for the Rheumatism," *The Gentleman's Magazine* (June 1, 1766): 280.

19 For more on this practice of recording newspaper recipes in family manuscripts, see Leong, *Recipes for Everyday Knowledge*, 147–72 and Katherine Allen, "Newspaper Remedies and Commercial Medicine in Eighteenth-Century Recipe Books," *The Recipes Project*, January 4, 2014.

20 Benjamin Franklin's *Poor Richard's Almanac* was retitled *Poor Richard Improved* in 1748, when Franklin took on David Hall as a partner in his publishing enterprises; the new version of the almanac continued to appear under Richard Saunders's name and grew longer (and more political). See William Pencak, "Politics and Ideology in *Poor Richard's Almanack*," *The Pennsylvania Magazine of History and Biography* 116, no. 2 (1992): 183–211. According to Labaree, Hall often oversaw the production and content of the almanacs when Franklin was engaged in public affairs, particularly during the years 1757–62. See Leonard W. Labaree, ed., *The Papers of Benjamin Franklin* (New Haven and London: Yale University Press, 1967), 12:3–4. In 1766, Franklin appeared before the House of Commons to plead for repeal of the 1765 Stamp Act, and he remained in England until 1775. See J. A. Leo Lemay, ed., *Benjamin Franklin: Writings* (New York: Library of America, 1987), 1484–87. As tempting as it is to see a connection between Franklin and the Frankland family, no such genealogical tie is readily apparent.

Even there, the recipe retains its "American" title, proclaiming a local origin to its Philadelphia audience even as its text remains remarkably close to the London printings, which Franklin may well have seen:

> The famous American Receipt for the Rheumatism
>
> Take of Garlic two cloves, of Gum
> Ammoniac one Drachm; blend them,
> by bruising together; make them into two
> or three Bolusses, with fair Water and swal-
> low them, one at Night, and one in the
> Morning. Drink, while taking this Recipe,
> Sassafras Tea, made very strong, so as to have
> the Tea-pot filled with Chips. This is ge-
> nerally found to banish the Rheumatism, and
> even Contraction in the Joints, in a very few
> times taking. It is very famous in *America*
> and an *Hundred Pounds* have been given for
> the Receipt.[21]

The Philadelphia almanac's seeming reliance on the printed London sources presents the "American" recipe as if it is unfamiliar to American readers. The text, after all, situates the writer as looking at America from afar, reporting on colonial behavior to those otherwise unaware of it.[22] This "famous" recipe, moreover, continued to cross oceans; by 1823, the cure had reached what is now Tasmania, where the *Hobart Town Gazette and Van Diemen's Land Advertiser* offered "the famous American receipt for the cure of the rheumatism, and, in some cases, even a contraction of the joints" to its readers, featuring the same ingredients, identical proportions, and largely similar language.[23]

21 Richard Saunders, *Poor Richard Improved* (Philadelphia, 1768). The recipe appears on the recto side of the two-page opening featuring September's forecasts. The edition features forecasts for the year 1769.

22 The recipe also appeared in another Philadelphia almanac in 1768, and no doubt in other printings in America as well. See Abraham Weatherwise, *Father Abraham's Almanack, for the Year of our Lord, 1769* (Philadelphia, 1768), [C3].

23 "Cure for the Rheumatism," *Hobart Town Gazette and Van Diemen's Land Advertiser* (September 20, 1823): 2. The "Famous American Receipt for Rheumatism," moreover, was not the only recipe for the ailment to claim roots in the western hemisphere. According to Katherine Allen, a recipe entitled "North American Prescription for Gout or Rheumatism," also "circulated widely in newspapers" and "appears often in recipe books"; its formulation proved remarkably

The notion of Carolina-born Lady Frankland copying a recipe from either a Philadelphia-printed almanac or a London newspaper, and retaining the label "American" in the process, suggests a perceived gap between herself and the colonies that had been her first home. Had she grown so distant from her roots that the recipe seemed to come from a different place? Or did it prompt a feeling of nostalgic connection, memories of the expertise of those administering successful rheumatism cures in her childhood surroundings? Perhaps the print format triggered a desire to copy the title with precision, even if that meant treating the recipe as if it came from a faraway place that she once had called home.

But perhaps the question about what makes this recipe "American" needs to be reframed. What if the recipe is considered American not because of its ingredients or the people who created it (whether colonists or Indigenous peoples), but because of the disease it treats? What if rheumatism itself, rather than the cure, is what makes this recipe "American"? Sassafras is undeniably sourced from the colonies, and, like all drugs, it was thought to cure diseases that thrived within its own habitat. If American plants cured the disease, then the disease itself would, logically, be linked to America too. Though rheumatism was certainly a concept in England before the establishment of transatlantic trade, the definition of the disease as commonly invoked in both print and manuscript began to transform after the founding of English colonies in North America. The recommended treatments changed in that process too, relying increasingly on imported ingredients. As more sassafras arrived in England, and its uses became more well known, one disease it treated—rheumatism—became a bigger concern in English culture, and its resident recipe manuscript keepers perceived an increased need to have cures at the ready. This conjunction signaled the success of an unarticulated but powerful colonial marketing coup, convincing the public to envision the affliction and the cure arriving on the same ships.

An American Affliction: Shifting Definitions of Rheumatism in an Age of Travel

"All countries have some peculiar diseases, arising from the climate, manner of living, occupations, predominant passions, and other causes, whose

different but equally American, containing "gum guaiacum, purified nitre, and Jamaican rum." See Katherine Allen, "Recipe Collections and the Realities of Fashionable Diseases in Eighteenth-Century Elite Domestic Medicine," *Literature and Medicine* 35, no. 2 (2017): 345.

separate and combined influence is but imperfectly known. In North America we may count five—nervous disorders, rheumatism, intermitting fevers, loss of teeth, and colds," declared Nicholas Collin, a Swedish clergyman who emersed himself in the study of natural history and culture upon his arrival in Philadelphia.[24] Though Collin never attained any particular scientific distinction, his remarks are, as Whitfield J. Bell puts it, "important precisely because so many others believed as he did" when he wrote his "An Essay on Those Inquiries in Natural Philosophy, Which at Present Are Most Beneficial to the United States of North America" in 1793.[25] And to him, rheumatism, like the suffering associated with seasoning, was a disease of *place*. Collin blamed the winter cold and poorly constructed houses whose fireplaces left "the fore part of the body ... almost roasted, while the back is freezing" for the prevalence of rheumatism in the Americas.[26] Jeremy Belknap used a similar rationale in describing the ailment's presence in New Hampshire, where "The chronic rheumatism is very common, but seldom proves mortal. It is often caused by the changes from heat to cold, to which people who labour and travel in all weathers, are exposed."[27] This inhospitable environment, however, could nonetheless provide the best cure. Collin urged American physicians "to substitute indigenous medicines of equal value for those imported, which by quantity or price cause a great national expense; and that are liable to adulteration, or depreciation by age." His explanation cites Indigenous sources without noting the specifics of their use, proclaiming, "The Indians have several remedies against the diseases and accidents arising from the climate, and their savage mode of life; as fevers, rheumatism, wounds, bruises, scalding, chillblains, [and] bite of venomous serpents," and he praises sassafras and several other local plants in particular for their power against rheumatism.[28]

24 Nicholas Collin, "An Essay on Those Inquiries in Natural Philosophy, which at Present are most Beneficial to the United States of North America," in "Nicholas Collin's Appeal to American Scientists," ed. Whitfield J. Bell, *William and Mary Quarterly* 13, no. 4 (1956): 525–50, esp. 525.
25 See Bell's introduction to Collin's "An Essay," 521. Bell reproduces the full text of Collin's "Essay" in the article. See Whitfield J. Bell, ed., "Nicholas Collin's Appeal to American Scientists," *William and Mary Quarterly* 13, no. 4 (1956): 519–50.
26 Collin, "An Essay," 528. Physicians and caregivers had long blamed environmental factors, such as cold and damp, for the condition; Greek physicians dating from Galen also attributed the affliction to an "innate predisposition" which made some individuals vulnerable to rheumatic symptoms throughout their lives. See Thomas G. Benedek, *Rheumatism: Its History from the Advent of Experimental Science to the Impact of Bacteriology* (New York: Nova Biomedical, 2017), 3.
27 Jeremy Belknap, *The History of New-Hampshire* (Boston: Belknap and Young, 1792), 3:232.
28 Collin, "An Essay," 538, 540.

Accessible records that focus on Indigenous accounts of rheumatism in North America are rare—something unsurprising given the many languages and oral traditions that have been overrun by the settler impulse to erase Indigenous experiences and knowledge. Virgil J. Vogel lists dozens of Indigenous cures for the condition labeled "rheumatism," though the term is loosely defined and his work covers more than four centuries.[29] He writes that early nineteenth-century accounts of the Quawpaw, Osage, and other tribes just west of the Mississippi revealed that "Rheumatism was a common ailment for which they used many methods of treatment."[30] William N. Fenton notes that, among the Iroquois, sassafras was "used in cases of rheumatism," but he does not specify the symptoms this treatment helped;[31] in the nineteenth century, Richard Foreman, identified as "a Cherokee doctor," prescribed sassafras for joint pain associated with the affliction, directing patients to "drink freely of the tea, and bathe the affected parts in tea of the same, until a high state of perspiration is produced, then wrap up warm in a blanket and cool off by degrees."[32] His work, transcribed by a white pharmacist, offers a Cherokee name for rheumatism as well—*Tsi-tah-nah-ler-la-skah*—and suggests that it "is quite frequent in the western country" and brought on by conditions often noted by European physicians such as "remaining too long on the damp grounds" or "being greatly heated and becoming suddenly cool."[33]

Europeans offer some tantalizing but nonspecific accounts of the disease as well during their earliest years in what has become Virginia. Many symptoms of the "terrible sort of gout" that the clergyman physician John Clayton encounters among Indigenous and English alike in the seventeenth-century Chesapeake resemble later discussions of rheumatism. After a severe initial fever, Clayton noted "those that seemeingly recover" suffered from "joynts [that] seem dislocated, & their hands utterly crippled."[34] Yet Clayton records no cures for this affliction. Though he

29 Virgil J. Vogel, *American Indian Medicine* (Norman: University of Oklahoma Press, 1970), 207–9.

30 Vogel, *American Indian Medicine*, 107.

31 William N. Fenton, *Contacts between Iroquois Herbalism and Colonial Medicine* (Seattle: Shorey Book Store, 1971), 517.

32 Richard Foreman and Jas. W. Mahoney, *The Cherokee Physician, or Indian Guide to Health* (Chapel Hill: University of North Carolina at Chapel Hill Library, 2018), 319–20.

33 Foreman, *The Cherokee Physician*, 71.

34 John Clayton, *The Reverend John Clayton: A Parson with a Scientific Mind*, ed. Edmund Berkeley and Dorothy Smith Berkeley (Charlottesville: Virginia Historical Society, 1965), 26, 4, 26. Interestingly, Benjamin Rush notes, "I have heard of two or three cases of the gout among the Indians, but it was only among those who had learned the use of rum, from the white people."

otherwise praises the tribes' resourcefulness with herbs, declaring that "every one according to his skill is a sort of Doctor as many women are in England,"[35] he records no attempts to treat this disease among either the Indigenous or the newly arrived English; in fact, he asks his English audience for potential cures.[36]

Rheumatism's definition in the period is difficult to settle on mostly because the collection of symptoms it encompassed, themselves tied to bodily fluids, continued to evolve and shift. Health issues associated with rheum, often described as rheumatic or labeled as rheumatism, had a long if indistinct history in England even before transatlantic travel became a cultural reality. Physicians and surgeons, relying on Galenic notions of the body, pictured rheum, or corrupt humors, accumulated in the head, resulting in fever or, in less dangerous cases, discharge from the eyes. Hence, Thomas Nashe could write of his ability to "rumatize my Readers eyes" when bringing them to tears.[37] Rheum could also cause dental pain. As Margaret Cavendish explains, "Tooth-aches are caused by Rheums: for the Rheum falling thereon, rots the Bones, or makes Holes therein; like as Water, continually dropping on a hard Stone, works a Passage thorow."[38]

In both manuscript and print, recipes for eliminating rheum from the head and chest suggest a conflation between rheum and mucous, conjuring images of head colds and flu. Just as some speak of colds moving from the head to chest today, early modern medical practitioners envisioned rheum descending from the head to the lungs, where it brought about breathing difficulties and coughing. Anne Brumwich's recipe manuscript, for example, contains "Another for the cough, & to dry upe *the* rume | & fleame."[39] James Hart's book *Klinike, or The Diet of the Diseased* contains a chapter vividly entitled "Of Snot or Snevell: Rheume falling downe upon the lungs and other pectorall parts."[40] Finally, when the concept of rheumatism had developed to encompass joint complaints, it was because rheum came to be seen as capable of sinking further through the body to create swelling in the lower extremities. In Roy Porter's words, "Like a traffic jam, a viscous rheum might

See Benjamin Rush, *An Oration, delivered February 4, 1774, before the American Philosophical Society, held at Philadelphia* (Philadelphia, 1774), 24.

35 Clayton, *The Reverend John Clayton*, 22.

36 Clayton, *The Reverend John Clayton*, 4.

37 Thomas Nash, *Christs Teares Over Ierusalem* (London, 1613), 56.

38 Margaret Cavendish, *The Worlds Olio* (London, 1655), 187.

39 Anne Brumwich, *Mrs Anne Brumwich her Booke of Receipts or Medicines for Severall Sores and other Infermities*, 1625, Wellcome MS 160, Wellcome Collection, London, England, 32.

40 James Hart, *Klinike, or The Diet of the Diseased* (London, 1633), 322.

snarl up around almost any organ."[41] Rheumatism's swollen joints lingered and recurred, and their chronic nature made their association with aging seems almost inevitable. Mrs. Corlyon, for example, identifies rheum as the reason for the geriatric suffering that Dr. Stevens's Water alleviates, going so far as to incorporate rheum into the title of the cure-all in her manuscript: "The making of Doctor Stephens water, it is good | for the Gowte, the Palsye the Toothache, and |for all diseases that come of Rhewme."[42]

The Practice of Physick—a 1655 English translation of Lazare Rivière's work credited to Nicholas Culpeper, Abdiah Cole, and William Rowland—attempts to clear up the confusion that inevitably occurred between gout and rheumatism. "This is no new Disease," the text proclaims of rheumatism, before declaring that Hippocrates and Galen both misunderstand it as misdirected blood causing "Inflamations" in "the fleshy Parts of the Body." The fault should not be seen in the blood but instead in what the text calls an "Inflamatory disposition, arising from fervor of the wheyish Humor" otherwise known as rheum.[43] In its earliest days, the fever that marked rheumatism's onset remained a chief characteristic, separating it from the localized joint pain of gout. Neither condition was seen as lethal; not until the nineteenth century did practitioners link the word *rheumatism* to the serious fevers that came to signal a life-threatening *rheumatic fever*.[44] In 1859, Alfred Baring Garrod proposed the term *rheumatoid arthritis* as a label for rheumatism's distinctive variety of joint pain; unhelpfully, he made that distinction in a treatise entitled *The Nature and Treatment of Gout and Rheumatic Gout*.[45] By the end of the nineteenth century, physicians began to question the term *rheumatism*'s usefulness and to urge it be abandoned as a diagnosis; those calls, coincidentally, emerged

41 Roy Porter and G. S. Rousseau, *Gout: The Patrician Malady* (New Haven: Yale University Press, 1998), 14.

42 Mrs. Corlyon, *A booke of such medicines as have been approved by the speciall practize of Mrs. Corlyon*, ca. 1606, Folger MS V.a. 388, Folger Shakespeare Library, Washington, DC, 160.

43 Lazare Rivière, *The Practice of Physick*, trans. Nicholas Culpeper, Abdiah Cole, and William Rowland (London 1655), 547–48.

44 W. S. C. Copeman, *A Short History of Gout and the Rheumatic Diseases* (Berkeley: University of California Press, 1964), 118. Peter C. English notes that "As a rule, in the eighteenth century, patients almost never died during an attack of rheumatism for any reason"—that is, until physicians in both London and Philadelphia began to notice a link between rheumatism and heart injury. See Peter C. English, *Rheumatic Fever in America and Britain: A Biological, Epidemiological, and Medical History* (New Brunswick, NJ: Rutgers University Press, 1999), 2.

45 See Alfred Baring Garrod, *The Nature and Treatment of Gout and Rheumatic Gout* (London, 1859), 526–56. For additional discussion, see English, *Rheumatic Fever in America and Britain*, 37. Also see "rheumatoid arthritis, n.," in *Oxford English Dictionary*, accessed July 18, 2023.

just as scientists were beginning to suggest a bacterial cause for rheumatic swelling.[46]

Despite these attempts to delineate the conditions, rheumatism overlapped with gout on both sides of the Atlantic well into the eighteenth century, and, perhaps unsurprisingly, perceptions of class made their way into these definitions. In England, Lord Chesterfield succinctly remarked, gout "is the distemper of a gentleman; whereas the rheumatism is the distemper of a hackney coachman or chairman, who is obliged to be out in all weathers."[47] In her study of eighteenth-century recipe manuscripts in England, Katherine Allen counts gout among the "fashionable" diseases, noting that the designation "did not necessarily refer to new diseases … but rather a newer rhetoric used to contextualize pre-existing ailments."[48] By 1724, such class-based distinctions were evident in English colonies as well, with Cotton Mather, in *The Angel of Bethesda*, labeling rheumatism "the Gout's younger brother" and further defining it as "a Bastard-Gout, [that] lies in wandring Pains of the Joints, which proceed … from a volatile Acid falling on the Membranes of them."[49]

This "wandring" was indeed the characteristic most settled on to mark the difference between the diseases: rheumatic pains moved throughout the body, while gout lingered in particular joints. Rheumatism, in short, traveled, while gout settled in to inflict persistent pain, usually in toes and knees. This distinction mattered to its sufferers as well. Gout, after all, was associated with the rich diets of the sedentary ruling classes, creating a further contrast with the colonial stock who ventured to foreign locales. Those inclined to cross the ocean, that is, experienced peripatetic rheumatism, with pains that traveled through the body in a seeming reflection of the sufferer's wanderlust.

Thomas Sydenham is credited with the first firm delineation of the difference between gout and rheumatism, emphasizing the affliction's trek through the sufferer's body in the process.[50] Translated from Latin into English in 1694, Sydenham's treatise describes rheumatism as an affliction

46 Benedek, *Rheumatism: Its History from the Advent of Experimental Science to the Impact of Bacteriology*, 13.

47 Philip Dormer Chesterfield, *The Letters of Philip Dormer Stanhope, 4th Earl of Chesterfield*, ed. Bonamy Dobrée (New York: AMS Press, 1932), 6:2685; I owe this reference to Porter and Rousseau, *Gout*, 50.

48 Allen, "Recipe Collections and the Realities of Fashionable Diseases," 335–36.

49 Cotton Mather, *Angel of Bethesda*, ed. Gordon W. Jones (Barre, VT: American Antiquarian Society, 1972), 135–36.

50 Copeman, *A Short History of Gout*, 121.

similar to the one Clayton noticed in Virginia, tracing its chronic joint pain back to a violent fever.

> In this Disease they are first taken with coldness and shivering, and the other symptoms of a Fever; and after a day or two (sometimes sooner) they are seiz'd with a most sharp pain, sometimes in one part and sometimes in another, but especially in the Wrists, Shoulders and Knees, which it leaves and assaults by turns, the part last affected remaining for some time after red and swoln. The Fever wears off by degrees, the pain still continuing, yea and sometimes raging more cruelly than before. In Rheumatic Aches of the Loins, there is a most violent pain that remains fix'd about the region of the Loins, and counterfeits the Stone; only the sick person is not troubled with a desire to vomit. He cannot lie in his Bed, but either leaps out of it, or sits upright in it, perpetually tossing his body backwards and forwards.[51]

Rheumatism not only moves from place to place within the body, it drives some sufferers into perpetual motion. His instructions for treatment, however, require no sassafras, even though those cures had already made their way into recipe manuscripts and other sources.[52] Instead, he prescribes a regimen of bleeding and bread poultices alongside herbal drinks made of lilies, purslane, lettuce, and syrup of violets. That said, he suggests that, should these treatments fail, practitioners turn to his section on scurvy, thus squarely associating rheumatism with the illness most associated with ocean crossings and colonial impulses.

Selling the Cure: Scurvy, Homegrown Rheum, and Traveling Rheumatism

The concept of rheumatism took root in English texts just as colonial expansion became a European pursuit. In 1538, Thomas Elyot included *Rheumatismus* in his dictionary, defining it clearly but unhelpfully as "the disease of rheume."[53] His listing of the term indicates that the word

51 Thomas Sydenham, *The Compleat Method of Curing Almost All Diseases* (London, 1694), 21.

52 Sydenham's book denotes only one occasion for sassafras, in a "Decoction for the Diet Drink" made largely of ingredients imported from the Americas (sarsaparilla roots, sassafras, China root, licorice, and anise). See Sydenham, *The Compleat Method of Curing Almost All Diseases*, 2.

53 Thomas Elyot, *The Dictionary of Syr Thomas Eliot Knight* (London, 1538), n.p.

was new to many, but the need to offer a definition suggests the diagnosis was becoming more common, either formally or informally. By the early seventeenth century, many recipes in domestic compilations grouped together rheumatism, gout, and sciatica, rarely making distinctions among the conditions. Lady Mary Jean Erskine, for example, devotes a "book" of her recipe manuscript—filling only half a page—to "diseases of the Joints & Rheumatick | pain of the whole body," but its first recipe is titled "of pain of the body called artritis | or the Gout."[54] Indeed, the initial symptoms of rheumatism could echo those of scurvy, leading Sydenham and other trained physicians to use the label *scorbutic rheumatism* as a diagnosis.[55] Such overlap in treatment and terminology situates rheumatism—a disease of traveling joint pain—alongside the long journeys associated with scurvy.

Though the two conditions featured similar lists of symptoms, scurvy and rheumatism unfolded according to different timelines. Rheumatism could be seen as stretching scurvy's myriad symptoms over a longer period, unfurling the disease's components—fevers, join pain, swelling, and tooth loss—in slow motion, to last a lifetime. Despite these efforts to draw distinctions among rheumatism, gout, and scurvy, practitioners of all stripes continued to discuss them together. In fact, the diseases grew so entangled that in 1684 Thomas Willis wrote "A long continued Gout very often joyns it to a Scurvy, and some Scorbutick affects [effects of scurvy] so plainly counterfeit the Gout that they cannot easily be distinguished." He continues to the confusing conclusion that, in these cases, the "Scorbutick affects which initiate the Gout are Rheumatism."[56] Even in the early seventeenth century, it is clear that antiscorbutic treatments—or anti-scurvy medicines, especially those effective against joint pain and tooth loss—were seen as also good for rheumatism. The compiler of one seventeenth-century recipe collection reveals a sense of this connection through her solid familiarity with medical language of the time, providing a list of many roots and herbs, from dock to

54 Erskine includes external and internal cures, stressing the use of dock root, wheat bran, and even puppies. She does not use sassafras, guaiacum, or sarsaparilla. See Lady Mary Jean Erskine, *The First Part of this Booke of Phisicke*, 1650–1700, University of Minnesota Libraries, MS Oversize WZ225 F527 1650, Owen H. Wangensteen Historical Library of Biology and Medicine, Minneapolis, MN, 26.

55 See Sydenham, *The Compleat Method of Curing Almost All Diseases*, 22. There, Sydenham recommends that if the usual bleeding and purging cures fail to help a rheumatic patient, "let him use the Antiscorbutic Electuary and Water describ'd in the Chapter of the Scurvy, which are also useful in the Scorbutic Rheumatism."

56 Thomas Willis, *The London Practice of Physick* (London, 1684), 497–98. Quoted in Thomas G. Benedek, *Rheumatism: Its History from Paleo-Pathology to the Advent of Experimental Science* (New York: Nova Biomedical, 2015), 64.

snakeroot, under the label "Antiscorbutics." The first herb listed is burdock, identified as a "remedy for Scrofula | or obstr[uction] of kidneys—good for Rheumatism [and] lepris Gout." Following it in the list is sarsaparilla, which is "good for Scrofula | or Rheumatism or such like affections."[57] The author of *Every Man his own Doctor* considered "slow fever," which he identifies as "the true Scorbutick fever," as among the most "difficult to manage" fevers; sassafras tea is key to its treatment.[58] Such classifications call on the perceived point of origin of rheumatism—the fever that occurs before the arrival of chronic joint point—and this invites a connection between transatlantic travel and the evolving understanding of rheumatism.

Sassafras, meanwhile, had been linked to scurvy from the earliest reports of its use among transatlantic travelers, when Indigenous women taught Jacques Cartier's expeditions the plant's properties. His 1535 accounts paint sassafras as the miracle cure for a plague affecting his crew that scholars have since labeled as scurvy. Its symptoms, unsurprisingly, blur with other conditions. In Hakluyt's printed account of Cartier's time in what is now Canada, sufferers "did lose all their strength, and could not stand on their feete, then did their legges swel, their sinnowes shrinke as blacke as any cole" and "their gummes [became] so rotten, that all the flesh did fall off, euen to the rootes of the teeth, which did also almost all fall out."[59] While these are classic scurvy symptoms, some of these afflictions—specifically the rotten teeth, swelling, and joint pain—came to be associated with rheumatic disfunctions.[60] Significantly, Edith Snook points out, Cartier credits God, not the Iroquois women who bring the cure, for providing the sassafras that treat the men's illness. Their leader Domagaia "sent two women to fetch some of it [sassafras leaves]" to make drink which cured the

57 In the same list, the collector praises roots of water dock for "clea[n]sing the Blood," a treatment that commonly involves sassafras. See *English Medicinal and Cookery Late 16th–mid-17th century*, 1540–1670, University of Minnesota Libraries WZ240 E58 1540, Owen H. Wangensteen Historical Library of Biology and Medicine, Minneapolis, MN, 35v.

58 *Every Man his own Doctor: or, The Poor Physician* (Williamsburg, 1736), 34.

59 Jacques Cartier, "A Shorte and Briefe Narration of the Navigation Made by the Commandment of the King of France, to the Islands of Canada," in *The Third and Last Volume of the Voyages, Navigations, Traffiques, and Discoveries of the English Nation*, ed. Richard Hakluyt (London, 1600), 226.

60 When the previously healthy 22-year-old sailor Philip Rougemont succumbed to the disease, Cartier ordered that he be autopsied (or at least "ripped" open) in hopes of further understanding the mysterious cause of his death. What they found was an inflamed heart, something that suggests an overlap with rheumatic fever. His swollen heart, accounts report, looked white, and, "when he was opened great quantitie of rotten blood issued out from about his heart." See Cartier, "A Shorte and Briefe Narration," 226.

Frenchmen's suffering, teaching them to "take the barke and leaues of the sayd tree, and boile them together, then to drinke of the sayd decoction euery other day, and to put the dregs of it upon his legs that is sicke." Cartier goes on to say that the Iroquois claimed the tree could "heale any other disease" before relating that "the tree is in their language called *Ameda* or *Hanneda*, this is thought to be the *Sassafras* tree."[61] Snook makes clear that ameda and sassafras are in fact distinct plants,[62] but the association between sassafras and the treatment of scurvy—and soon rheumatism—lingered, making the tree a valuable resource for both healthcare and commerce in the decades to come.

If scurvy is the disease of exploration—of seafaring and the initial sickness brought on by settling on unfamiliar shores—rheumatism is the disease of colonization, or the struggle to establish a long-term presence in a foreign environment. As Jonathan Lamb shows, the cause of scurvy was debated until the discovery of Vitamin C, but explorers and physicians alike knew that it struck after about three months away from port, when fresh food from home ran out.[63] As people ventured further from home, they tested their physical limits, not only through the ordeals of travel but, in their minds, by leaving behind the airs, waters, and places that had shaped their bodily constitutions. Lamb argues that scurvy is not merely the "disease of discovery"; it is in the broader picture "a disease of motion and displacement, the pathology of imperial expansion, in which home stands as the norm from which ambitious nations cause their servants to deviate."[64] In that process, travelers imposed insurmountable distance between themselves and the natural environments that best sustained—and, when necessary, repaired—their health. Rheumatism in the logic of the time stretches out this suffering, tracing a long-term impact of this movement away from home. This exposure to the climates of other lands invites a connection between transatlantic travel and the evolving understanding of rheumatism; the damage done by disconnection lingers, even upon return to one's homeland. Casting rheumatism as an American disease thus marks the affected body's association with displacement and life on foreign shores.

61 Cartier, "A Shorte and Briefe Narration," 227.

62 Snook points out that Cartier's identification of the cure as sassafras was likely not correct, given that the tree does not grow in the northerly location he describes. She suggests that the tree was in fact ameda. See Snook, "Grace Mildmay's Recipes and Indigenous Knowledge," 224–25.

63 Jonathan Lamb, *Scurvy: The Disease of Discovery* (Princeton: Princeton University Press, 2017), 75–76.

64 Lamb, *Scurvy*, 7, 22.

Jamestown, Seasoning, and Sassafras

While Europeans sailed westward in hopes of finding resources to sell back home, they often found themselves searching first for cures to local illnesses they encountered upon arrival. When they landed, after all, they had already encountered unhealthy conditions onboard ship, subsisting on preserved foods that left them at risk of scurvy and other forms of dietary deficiency. Once off the boats, they encountered water and foods to which their bodies were not accustomed, if such provisions were available at all. The arrival of additional settlers at Jamestown, for example, exacerbated food scarcity in the colony, contributing to an increase in scurvy. This experience of hunger only heightened the physical and mental stress of the seasoning period. As Martha Robinson points out, English colonists were predisposed to worry about their ability to adjust to these surroundings, since they "believed that their bodies were peculiarly suited to cold, moist lands and could not easily endure the heat of Spain, the West Indies, or Virginia."[65] The process of "seasoning," as discussed in the previous chapter, could certainly be arduous, even if it left those who survived buffered against the environmental hazards of the unfamiliar surroundings. But, thanks to earlier Spanish and French reports of Indigenous treatments for the fevers and illnesses lurking in the Americas, some English settlers arrived armed with knowledge for easing the process of seasoning—and sassafras was key to those efforts. More curious, some of the particulars of seasoning in the Americas encompassed the symptoms that later came to be grouped together under the label of rheumatism.

Seasoning and sassafras were linked from the tree's first appearance in a European medical text. However, the Spanish merchant Nicolás Monardes, credited with the first accounts of sassafras in 1565, and his English translator John Frampton showed little interest in the people who informed Europeans of the plant's power to lessen fever. Instead, Monardes talks about American plants with, in Bleichmar's words, the "manic enthusiasm of the advertising pitch"[66] —something that betrays his intent to generate a market for these

65 Martha K. Robinson, "New Worlds, New Medicines: Indian Remedies and English Medicine in Early America," *Early American Studies: An Interdisciplinary Journal* 3, no. 1 (2005): 98.
66 Bleichmar, "Books, Bodies, and Fields," 96. Frampton's approach likely stems from his own interest in gleaning profit from New World trade, raising awareness of products available through the newly formed Spanish Company which was backed by his patron Edward Dyer, Earl of Leicester. See Donald Beecher, "John Frampton of Bristol: Trader and Translator," in *Travel and Translation in the Early Modern Period*, ed. Carmine G. Di Biase (Amsterdam: Rodopi, 2006), 106–7. In a later article, Beecher even proclaims "The point must not be belaboured, but through

imports.[67] When Spaniards began to suffer from the tropical environment, Monardes explained, they turned as they had been taught, by sources never explicitly named, to sassafras, which provided great relief.

> Our Spaniards began to cure themselues with the water of this Tree, and it wrought in them great effectes, that are almost incredible: for with the naughtie meates & drinking of the rawe waters, & sleeping in the dewes, the most parte of them fell into continuall Agues, of the which many of them came into opilations, and from the opilations they began to swell, and when the euil came first, immediatly it began to take away the lust that they had to their meate, and then happened to them other accidents, and diseases, as such like Feuers are accustomed to bring.[68]

Sassafras provided near-immediate relief for seasoning's fever, but not all symptoms disappeared so quickly. Monardes does not immediately link "opilations" to persistent joint problems, nor does he explicitly associate them with problems stemming from the flow of rheum within the body. That said, he twice mentions mobility problems that the climate brings, and that sassafras can counter. Many "that bee lame or creeples, and in them that are not able to goe, nor to moue themselues," he writes, have been healed by taking sassafras tea "hot in the morning, and procuring sweate all that hee can, eating things of diet, and drinking the simple water continually."[69]

When John Frampton's English translation of Monardes's work became available in 1580, it inspired Thomas Hariot and others like him to consider

Frampton's offices, in bringing Monardes to the attention of English readers, and in converting this Spanish pharmaceutical scripture into an English one, there may be seen the foundation for incentives behind the English colonization of Virginia on the basis of commodities formerly little to be imagined." See Donald Beecher, "Nicolás Monardes, John Frampton and the Medical Wonders of the New World," in *Humanismo e ciência: Antiguidade erenascimento*, eds. António Manuel Lopes Andraade, Carlos de Miguel Mora, and João Manuel Nunes Torrão (Coimbra: Imprensa da Universidade de Coimbra, 2015), 148.

67 What's more, this dissociation of American plants from the Indigenous peoples who introduced them to Europeans highlights a typical colonial pattern of domination. Passing on knowledge of the lifesaving sassafras root, ironically, only caused suffering for those providing the cure. As Clare Griffin emphasizes, "we are looking at Europeans appropriating and profiting from expertise on sassafras root as an anti-febrile, while simultaneously killing the Timucua and other Native American experts on American medicinal flora, whose knowledge was the very basis of all subsequent ideas about and uses of sassafras." Griffin, "Disentangling Commodity Histories," 3. The French did not fare too well in this particular case either.

68 Nicolás Monardes, *Ioyfull Newes Out of the New-found Worlde*, trans. John Frampton (London, 1580), 46v.

69 Monardes, *Ioyfull Newes Out of the New-found Worlde*, 52v.

sassafras as a potentially marketable natural resource. In fact, Sir Walter Ralegh established the colony at Roanoke largely because of its plentiful sassafras, and he had to struggle to retain his monopoly as other expeditions brought in imports of the wood from New England.[70] No wonder later colonists foresaw the tree's potential value for sustaining the Jamestown venture. The trees were so plentiful that their scent was said to reach ships well before they approached shore,[71] and they were already growing, when other marketable plants like tobacco required careful (and not always successful) cultivation.[72] In fact, the first letter ever written from Jamestown wondered at the plentiful sassafras, reporting they had already harvested "two tunnes at least" while also expressing concern that sending too much of it back would "pull down our price for a long time."[73] Regardless, the Virginia Company instructed the Jamestown authorities in 1610 to send sassafras root back to London to meet consistent consumer demand.[74] Sassafras soon regularly filled the holds of vessels sailing eastward, where it was valued for its scent as well as its medicinal properties.[75]

And sassafras did indeed find a market in England, appearing in home recipe manuscripts early in the 1600s. Frances Catchmay and Lady Grace Mildmay

70 For accounts of sassafras voyages in what is now New England—one by Captain Bartholomew Gilbert and Captain Bartholomew Gosnold in 1602 and another by a rogue investors' group led by Martin Pring in 1603, see Holly Dugan, *The Ephemeral History of Perfume: Scent and Sense in Early Modern England* (Baltimore: Johns Hopkins University Press, 2011), 89–90, 92 and Graham Roebuck, "Sassafras," in *The Mysterious and the Foreign in Early Modern England*, eds. Helen Ostovich and Mary V. Silcox (Newark: University of Delaware Press, 2008), 172–73.

71 Dugan suggests that other trees furnished part of the smell, quoting Philip Amadas and Arthur Barlowe as finding their ship in "the midst of some delicate garden abounding with all kinds of odoriferous flowers" as they approached the Carolinas in 1584; see Dugan, *The Ephemeral History of Perfume*, 72.

72 "Groves of large sassafras trees grew in abundance in the English North American colonies, but as their roots and bark were stripped the trees died back, creating a boom-bust cycle in exports of sassafras," Maydom observes. See Katrina Elizabeth Maydom, "New World Drugs in England's Early Empire," PhD diss., (Cambridge University, 2018), 84. Dugan reports the Jamestown settlers were unable to meet their quotas of gathered sassafras by 1622; see Dugan, *The Ephemeral History of Perfume*, 93.

73 Wyndham Bolling Blanton, *Medicine in Virginia in the Seventeenth Century* (New York: Arno Press, 1972), 108–9; quoting Mary Newton Stanard, *The Story of Virginia's First Century* (Philadelphia: Lippincott, 1928), 40.

74 Philip Alexander Bruce, *Economic History of Virginia in the Seventeenth Century* (London: Macmillan, 1896), 261–62.

75 For a history of European sassafras harvesting and shipping in the Americas, see Russell M. Magnaghi, "Sassafras and Its Role in Early America, 1562–1662," *Tera Incognitae* 29, no. 1 (1997): 10–21. Maydom offers tables showing trends in "New World Drugs in England's Early Empire." Also see Dugan, *The Ephemeral History of Perfume*, 73–76.

included sassafras in their collections, in pages that Edith Snook dates to before 1625.[76] Both compilers use sassafras for syphilis—itself seen as an imported disease, potentially linked to America—and often combine the root with other American ingredients like sarsaparilla, on the theory that plants from the disease's homeland make the best cures. Before 1650 then, sassafras had, in Snook's words, "become part of an English culture of intellectual exchange, among women, scholars, physicians, families, and acquaintances."[77]

Evolving Treatment for Traveling Pains: Rheumatism in Manuscript Recipes

The recipes aiming to treat rheumatism in manuscript recipe collections, meanwhile, offer a glimpse of compilers struggling to grasp the slippery disease. Rheumatism proved hard to pin down, despite compilers' efforts to capture the condition in writing. A seventeenth-century manuscript at the University of Pennsylvania, for example, contains three cures for rheumatism, each vastly different from the other. The first entry in this English collection reflects the compiler's struggle to spell the condition's name, first writing "reuatism," then backtracking to insert an *m*, and then scratching most of the word out to replace it with "reumatism."[78] Though such corrections often happen in these manuscripts, this instance suggests the writer is thinking phonetically as she works to capture a challenging, unfamiliar word. It is also certainly striking that the manuscript's first cure incorporates many American plants. In fact, the recipe requires a hodge podge of American ingredients, seeming to throw in everything the New World has to offer in hopes that they can provide relief for a seemingly American disease.

> Mrs Allibons ressett for a re[m]uatism reumatism.
>
> Take a quarter of a pound of Sasaparella a quarter of a pound of Sasafras[,] of China, Lignum vita and hartshorne of each 2 ounces, one ounce of

76 See Lady Frances Catchmay, *A Booke of Medicens*, seventeenth century, Wellcome MS 1841a, Wellcome Collection, London, England, 46, and Edith Snook, "English Women's Writing and Indigenous Medical Knowledge in the Early Modern Atlantic World," in *A History of Early Modern Women's Writing*, ed. Patricia Phillippy (Cambridge: Cambridge University Press, 2018), 391–93.
77 Snook, "English Women's Writing and Indigenous Medical Knowledge in the Early Modern Atlantic World," 395.
78 *Recipe Book*, 1663, University of Pennsylvania Ms. Codex 252, University of Pennsylvania, Philadelphia, PA, 231.

> Licorish; Caraway Seed, and sweet fenell seeds, of eache half an ounce
> halfe a pound of raisons of the sun, put it into 14 quarts of Spring watter
> lett it stand all night Close covered the next day Sett it one a slow fire let
> it simmer 24 hours ten straine it through a musline, take of
> this warme half a pint morning and night
>
> put 7 quarts of watter upon the same drugs lett them stew 12 hours
> drink this when ever you are a drye and noe other drinke for a
> month.[79]

Relying on sarsaparilla, sassafras, and guaiacum (here referred to as Lignum vita), the recipe is a conglomeration of American ingredients. The writer never explicitly states the origins for rheumatism itself, yet its use of so many imports from the other side of the Atlantic recalls the key biological principles of colonial health: that specific environments contain the cures for the illnesses most commonly found there. Even China root participates in this local logic, given that it was often harvested in the Americas as well.[80] This same manuscript, however, contains two other cures for rheumatism, neither of which involves any American ingredients whatsoever. "Mrs. Briscoes ressett for a rumetisme," for example, recommends a mustard plaster followed by bleeding, if necessary, and a later hand records "A Recipe to Cure the Rumatism" that calls for apples, sherry, and antimony.[81] These recipes exhibit a variety of possible approaches to treatment, highlighting the evolving perceptions of the condition, its symptoms, and its perceived causes (as well as of its spelling).

Domestic recipe manuscripts in England continued to emphasize American ingredients in compounds used to counter rheumatism, often combining several imported plants in their efforts. University of Pennsylvania Ms. Codex 1038, written in England between 1765 and 1830, records a recipe by Mrs. Hayes for "Rheumatism & Cramp" that requires carefully measured amounts of guaiacum, balsam of Peru, and rum.[82] Other recipes, however, combine imported American ingredients with those from more local sources. Mary Baumfylde, in the early eighteenth century, relies on "half an ounce of Gumgoacum | steept in half a pint of best | brandy" in her cure "For the

79 *Recipe Book*, 1663, University of Pennsylvania Ms. Codex 252, 231.

80 See Magnaghi, "Sassafras and Its Role in Early America, 1562–1662," 17.

81 *Recipe Book*, 1663, University of Pennsylvania Ms. Codex 252, 253, 268.

82 *Recipe Book*, 1765, University of Pennsylvania Ms. Codex 1038, University of Pennsylvania, Philadelphia, PA, 160.

Rheumatism."[83] A seventeenth-century miscellany associated with Edmund Fettiplace and his family, meanwhile, contains nine different recipes for rheumatism cures. These recipes all illustrate a sustained confusion between rheumatism and gout, and they aim toward inclusiveness in that, if the compiler imagined even a slim possibility of the cure's usefulness for a condition, that condition would be named in the recipe. The first, under the heading "for the Gout, Rheumatism or sciatica," speaks primarily of gout, advising a tincture of red wine and cochineal and noting, "If you have the Rheumatism or | sciatica, take the Tincture as before | but in a larger Quantity."[84] The second recipe, "A Dyet Drink for the Rheumatism," combines local and American ingredients with abandon, mixing sassafras, guaiacum, and senna with dock root and ground ivy.[85] Further into the collection's pages, as rheumatism is referenced more frequently, English plants reassert themselves into the recipes, suggesting that rheumatism had planted itself firmly in the country's list of routine ailments.

Combinations of sassafras with other American ingredients certainly occurred in rheumatism recipes used in settler homes as well. Perhaps surprisingly given its association with cold, such rheumatism recipes in manuscript appear with great frequency in collections linked to regions between the mid-Atlantic and the Carolinas.[86] An insertion into Ellen Fitzhugh's eighteenth-century book, from America's middle Atlantic, creates a sassafras tea very much like "The Famous American Receipt for the Rheumatism" in the Frankland manuscript:

> Mrs. Raper's Receipt for the
> Rhuematism
>
> Sacafras the Chips & Bark
> Peruvian Bark grosly Powderd
> Guaicom Chips

83 Mary Baumfylde, *Medicinal and Cookery Recipes of Mary Baumfylde*, 1626, Folger MS V.a. 456, Folger Shakespeare Library, Washington, DC, 69v.

84 *Miscellany*, 1613, Folger MS V.a. 260, Folger Shakespeare Library, Washington, DC, 11r–11v.

85 *Miscellany*, 1613, Folger MS V.a. 260, 15r.

86 Walden suggests that manuscript recipe culture itself lingered longer in this region. See Sarah Walden, *Tasteful Domesticity: Women's Rhetoric and the American Cookbook, 1790–1940* (Pittsburgh: University of Pittsburgh Press, 2018), 83–84. Cromwell incorporates cures for gout but not rheumatism in her Massachusetts-based manuscript, though she uses sassafras "to cleans & purifie the bloud," and to cure scurvy. See Charles Brigham, *Account Book [manuscript]*, 1650–1730s, American Antiquarian Society, Folio Vols. B, American Antiquarian Society, Worcester, MA, 73, 96.

Buckbearn, nicely dry'd
of each an eaqual quanty made
into Tea pretty strong to be
taken a little warm twice
a Day aboute half a Pint
each time.[87]

The recipe incorporates additional American botanical materials, in a way that mirrors the methods of English manuscript books and may reflect hopes that overwhelming the disease with treatment would do the trick. Eliza Pinckney of South Carolina also offers multiple recipes for rheumatism in her eighteenth-century recipe manuscript; the first is a combination of herbal oils combined with tobacco and rosemary, stuffed in a pipe and smoked, and notes included at the end of her book offer three recipes for the condition that use guaiacum.[88] A later American collection offers a cure "To make a Bath, and Poultice for [a] sore Leg" which does not directly invoke rheumatism in its title but which uses ingredients common to the disease's cures, calling for "Bark of Sassafras Root, Poke root, Spicewood bark, | red-willow bark, and white oak bark" stewed together.[89] In Nova Scotia, meanwhile, Sarah Creighton Wilkins includes a tea of sassafras, sarsaparilla, and guaiacum in her recipe "For the Rheumatism" in 1814.[90]

Other rheumatism cures in American collections, however, hint at more complicated underlying ideas of the condition's origins by invoking English medical traditions. That is, some American recipes for rheumatism call for ingredients that would be imported to America, rather than harvested from local soils. In the case of Jane Randolph's 1743 manuscript, compiled in Virginia, two recipes illustrate the conflicting identities—and accompanying assumptions about connection to environment and bodily health—that colonists experienced. The first, "Baron's Receipt for a Rumatism," reflects notions of the disease as an internal condition lingering from a fever, directing users to "Put 4 oz: of Gumgoacum into a quart of Rum" and take

87 Ellen Fitzhugh, *Manuscript Recipe Book*, 1842, University of Pennsylvania Ms. Codex 651, University of Pennsylvania, Philadelphia, PA, 65. The recipe is on an unnumbered page inserted into the bound collection. While this insertion has no date, other insertions into the collection date from the early nineteenth century.

88 Eliza Pinckney, *Receipt Book Kept by Eliza L. Pinckney*, 1756, South Carolina Historical Society MS 43-2178, Lowcountry Digital Library, Charleston, SC, 13, 47.

89 *Cookery and Medicinal Receipts*, 1820, University of Minnesota MS Small QV C773 1820, Owen H. Wangensteen Historical Library of Biology and Medicine, Minneapolis, MN, 15.

90 Sarah Creighton Wilkins, "For the Rheumatism," *Early Modern Maritime Recipes*.

a spoonful each morning and evening; the second, "For the Rheumatism," immediately follows on the page and calls for a concoction of cochineal and English saffron, to be both taken internally and used as an external treatment for pained joints.[91] The first relies on materials associated with the Western hemisphere, calling on rum and guaiacum imported but readily available from the sources not too far south of Virginia's ports. The second, however, depends on an explicitly English herb, combined with cochineal, an import from colonies located further away in the Americas.

The causes of rheumatism are themselves fluid—the disease, after all, can be traced to the motions of liquidy rheum. It is perhaps fitting, then, that in its increasingly common appearances in recipe manuscripts in the eighteenth century rheumatism proves ill-defined but also strangely convenient. The term accommodated a wide array of symptoms, and its use may reflect its easy application as well as its murky boundaries in relation to conditions like gout and sciatica. At the same time, discussions of and treatments for rheumatism reflect a movement away from its febrile origins, emphasizing instead the wandering joint pains that linger for years beyond the condition's onset. This deemphasis of fever as the condition's first symptom severs rheumatism's early connections to scurvy, a disease that carried with it resonances of transatlantic travel and its dangers. Similarly, this diminishing role of fever also lessened the lingering echoes of seasoning that might otherwise accompany rheumatism.

Rheumatism and colonial trade thus worked together to interfere with established narratives about the connections between places and the diseases that they were seen as nurturing. The era's growing trade networks allowed sufferers from either side of the Atlantic to find cures, often skirting the geographic challenges that earlier limited the flow of goods from abroad that could best treat the affliction. These same networks also obscured the Indigenous sources of medical knowledge, allowing trade itself to stand in the popular mindset as the origin of new cures. While English colonial travels enabled home practitioners to mingle together ingredients from different lands to make rheumatism cures, rheumatism itself had the notably ironic effect of impeding the physical movement of those who suffered from the ailment. The mobility of medicinal compounds also suggested that people from different places could react in similar ways to botanical cures, even though this violated Hippocratic principles of the interplay between diseases, bodies, and environment. The result, clearly visible in

91 Katherine E. Harbury, *Colonial Virginia's Cooking Dynasty* (Columbia: University of South Carolina Press, 2004), 416.s

early modern recipe manuscripts, was a new flexibility in the classical *Airs, Waters, Places* tradition—a flexibility that allowed English household cures to adjust to new environments, ready to meet new conditions, both at home and abroad, as they encountered them.

Epilogue: The Travels of the Great Cordial

Abstract: Recipe manuscripts illustrate their compilers' habits for recording knowledge, yet they rarely offer the complete picture today's readers might crave. This chapter explores how early modern practitioners and modern scholars alike have read one of Sir Walter Ralegh's most significant recipes alongside writings recounting his travels and political troubles. The details available regarding this recipe, however, offer little clarification of its origins. The Great Cordial's extensive ingredient list, incorporating materials from all over the globe, continued to evolve after Ralegh's death, as domestic compilers and the era's famous scientists worked to understand the recipe and its properties. The recipe's domestic creation and use, I argue, retains a sense of the inscrutable, despite the details supplied for its creation.

Keywords: Robert Boyle; Walter Ralegh; Sandys family; Katherine Jones, Lady Ranelagh; Indigenous knowledge

Travel and trade in the seventeenth century changed the domestic healthcare practices found in English manuscript recipe books, leading to the incorporation not just of new ingredients but of new ideas of disease and its cures. Just as importantly, travel also altered the ways that people perceived the impact of environment on their bodies. Everyday English people of the era increasingly took up longer journeys, venturing to nearby cities and country retreats if not to lands across the ocean. The growing certainty with which they could complete these journeys, moreover, changed their perceptions of their danger. The English were testing their physical limits, not only through the ordeals of travel but, in their minds, by leaving behind the airs, waters, and places that had shaped their bodily constitutions. In that process, they often imposed substantial, and at times even insurmountable, distance between themselves and the natural environments they had long

Nunn, Hillary M. *Recipes on the Move in Early Modern England and British North America: Domestic Medicine, Mobility, and Manuscript Culture*. Amsterdam: Amsterdam University Press, 2025.
DOI 10.5117/9789463723398_EPI

envisioned as the root of their health. They also remained sure that their new surroundings would contain the appropriate cures for their recovery should they fall ill. In some ways, the changes of environment that came with such mobility cast doubt on the usefulness of bringing recipe manuscripts along on these journeys. Like the people who first wrote in them, most of these manuscript collections were shaped by their English surroundings, incorporating area plant life, animals, and water sources, as well as local healthcare knowledge and practices. They, along with the bodies of their owners, would need to change upon reaching their destinations in order to function effectively.

The effects of these changed environments as manifested in manuscript collections, however, often proved subtle, if they were visible at all. Most recipe manuscripts of the era are accretive documents, incorporating new materials with the passage of time, and, while compilers often made notes on recipes written in their books' earlier pages, the habit of crossing out entries is relatively rare. This may signal that users seldom consulted the pages filled years earlier, something that repetition of identical recipes within the same manuscript suggests. At the same time, these earlier pages constitute an archive of previous practices, ones that family members could see as evidence of their forebears' connection to their own environments and each other. Crossing out recipes written by earlier generations would amount to severing family connections, not just to those recipe keepers but to the lands they lived on, the healthcare traditions that sustained them, and the local ingredients that nurtured their bodies. Perpetuating such connections could explain why so many compilers copied out the recipe for Dr. Stevens's Water, with or without its seemingly impossible claims for long life. Suggesting the possibility of bodily longevity at home in England, the cordial offered glimmers of hope to those facing less friendly environments in the American colonies—if not for themselves, for those to follow.

In this sense, recipes play a role in European settler colonialism, showing the arriving population how to stay put and stay well in new lands. Edith Snook offers one memorable example, in the form of a recipe for roofing material, supposedly sent from the Royal Society of Sweden to the Royal Society in London, that purports to have created roofs that "stood in Sweden above a century, and still want no repair." The recipe appeared in a Nova Scotia newspaper in 1799, after appearing in Charleston in 1796 and working its way up the North American coastline. The recipe "may seem innocent," Snook observes, "but its writer, despite not being overtly engaged in political polemic, was claiming authority from European royal societies while houses built for a hundred years were structures for claiming sovereignty and for coming to stay."[1] At the same time, such recipes were on the move, working their way through the communication channels that connected colonies to one another and to the European continent. They insisted that European knowledge could be deployed in new settings—that familiarity with Swedish roofing could be of use in places ranging from London, to South Carolina, to Nova Scotia, despite the drastically different climates in these locations—and that it could root Europeans in their new homes in the process. As Snook points out, knowledge communicated through the recipe form allowed later settlers to bring European "ways of knowing to the western side of the Atlantic and to avoid the engagement and learning from Indigenous peoples that had been so necessary to their survival when they first arrived."[2]

Manuscript recipe books, even when uprooted from their initial homes, thus brought a sense of security to those adjusting to new environments, keeping their bodies connected to the places they left and preventing them from feeling fully part of the alien lands they came to occupy. The formation of English households in America nonetheless underwent adjustments to thinking about the relationship between human bodies and their environments. The long-held Galenic ideas that people are healthiest in the environments of their birth—and that this connection to place dominated the individual body's constitution—could not withstand the pressure of expansionist desires, and the realities of colonial life. Not only did people travel to far-off locations and encounter new diseases and new medicinal plants; they took what they found back to England and to European markets for use by people otherwise disconnected from American environments. Of course, these trade patterns had long been in existence in England, illustrated by the many imported ingredients that permeated Ann Fanshawe's recipe book even before she left on her most-noted travels. As the influx of goods from abroad led to further saturation of the English markets, the notion that healthcare treatments should, ideally, spring from the same environments that caused illnesses, or at least nurtured them, gradually eroded as more ingredients from abroad became available. This turn to American ingredients, moreover, highlighted the increasing impression that changes to English health, as evidenced through diseases like rheumatism, originated from the western side of the Atlantic.

1 Edith Snook, "The Recipes of Jonathan Odell and 18th-Century Settler Colonialism in the Maritimes," *Acaciensis* 49, no. 2 (2020): 122.

2 Snook, "The Recipes of Jonathan Odell," 126.

Manuscript Manifestations of Ralegh's Great Cordial

Tracing the strands that intertwine in "The Great Cordial"—a complicated cure-all linked to Sir Walter Ralegh—reinforces the fact that it is not just ingredients that travel; recipes themselves cover a great deal of ground, appearing in different places, and in different forms, as people share them and copy them into their own manuscript collections. In some ways, the Great Cordial may seem unlike many recipes found in domestic recipe manuscripts in that it comes with a written creation story attached to a famous explorer. The recipe's pedigree, however, lends the cure little textual stability;[3] in fact, as we will see, the recipe itself appears in at least one manuscript without the Ralegh name that allegedly bestows its greatness upon it. The recipe's complexity and alchemical leanings too set it apart from many cures in domestic manuscripts. Few domestic recipes, after all, earned discussion among respected scientists in print treatises, as the Great Cordial does. King Charles II even commanded that one of these scientists, Dr. Nicaise Le Fèbure, explain the recipe's workings at a public demonstration at court in September of 1662. John Evelyn notes that he accompanied the king to see the "accurate preparation for the composing [of] Sir Walter Raleigh's rare cordial," where Le Fèbure made a "learned discourse ... in French on each ingredient."[4] Two years later, in 1664, Le Fèbure published his annotation of the Great Cordial's ingredients in a 110-page pamphlet.[5] Meanwhile, in 1663, Sir Robert Boyle pointedly included a much briefer recipe for the Great Cordial in *Some Considerations Touching the Vsefulnesse of Experimental Naturall Philosophy*. "I am induc'd," he asserts, "to annex here the yet unpublish'd Receipt, partly, because there are divers Receipts that are each pretended to be the true, magnify'd by their several Possessors." Boyle more than insist his version is genuine; he rests his claim on his purported access to a Ralegh family manuscript, noting that he "had the liberty of looking it out in a Receipt Book, preserved by the Authors

3 This instability is heightened by the existence of a second cordial recipe, sometimes called a cordial jelly, associated with Ralegh. Praised for its aid to digestion, this recipe involves strawberries and a great deal of sugar. See, for example, "An Excellent Coridal jelly a Comforter of the harte & helpe | to digesture of sir walter raleigh," *A Book of Receipts, which was Given me by Several Men for Several Causes, Griefs and Diseases*, c. 1625–c. 1700, Folger MS V.a.361, Folger Shakespeare Library, Washington, DC, 38r.

4 John Evelyn, *The Diary and Correspondence of John Evelyn, F.R.S*, ed. William Bray (London, 1857), 1:368–69.

5 Nicaise Le Fèbure, *A Discourse upon Sr Walter Rawleigh's Great Cordial*, (London, 1664).

Son."[6] Yet, even as the Great Cordial made its way to the Boyle family's elite scientific circles, it also appears in manuscript collections that have no obvious connection to this privileged realm, where it sometimes flaunts its pedigree and other times does not.

Ironically, while Ralegh's long association with transatlantic voyages contributed an American aura to the Great Cordial recipe, explanations of its creation owe much to his time of isolation in a distinctly English spot: the Tower of London, where he was held between 1603 and 1617. Ralegh was briefly released from captivity to undertake a last journey to Guiana, but was nonetheless executed upon his return in 1618. During his time in the Tower, Ralegh converted a chicken coop into a still room and conducted experiments using plants from the Tower garden.[7] He managed to acquire imported ingredients as well, producing a Balsam of Guiana that Madame de Beaumont, wife of the French ambassador, credited with saving her life, and which Queen Anne mistakenly hoped would save the ailing heir Prince Henry in 1612.[8] That medicine's title proclaims its direct connection to an American source—the land of Guiana where Ralegh hoped to leave his mark—leading Charles Nicholl, among others, to conclude that the balsam could be a version of the Great Cordial recipe, which also specifically demands another American ingredient: sassafras from Virginia.

Nicholl's admission that this connection is "plausible but unprovable"[9] highlights the slipperiness that accompanies even the most documented of recipe histories. Locating Ralegh's experiments in the Tower creates a more controlled environment for them, establishing a domestic still room in a closely circumscribed location, one under heavy surveillance at that. Such close quarters might conjure images of Ralegh working alone while singlehandedly shaping the medicines produced under his name. But to

6 Robert Boyle, *Some Considerations Touching the Vsefulnesse of Experimental Naturall Philosophy* (Oxford, 1663), 316.

7 For more on the history of the recipe, see John Knott, "Sir Walter Raleigh's 'Royal Cordial,'" *Dublin Journal of Medical Science* 121 (1906): 63–70, 131–43, and Charles Nicholl, *The Creature in the Map: A Journey to El Dorado* (Chicago: University of Chicago Press, 1995), 278–87. Shirley, after consulting manuscripts detailing expenses associated with the Tower still room, concludes that, though Ralegh and his compatriots produced various liquors, "there is little or no evidence of any wide-scale experimentation in either chemistry as we know it, or in alchemy." See John William Shirley, "The Scientific Experiments of Sir Walter Ralegh, the Wizard Earl, and the Three Magi in the Tower 1603–1617," *Ambix* 4, no. 1–2 (1949): 63. Gallay provides an introduction to the Great Cordial's story as well, in Alan Gallay, *Walter Ralegh: Architect of Empire* (New York: Basic, 2019), 430–40.

8 Nicholl, *The Creature in the Map*, 282.

9 Nicholl, *The Creature in the Map*, 287.

see Ralegh as a solitary presence in an otherwise unoccupied space is as inaccurate as imagining him sailing without help to an empty American continent. He had at least one assistant on site, who attended him for twelve years and later worked as a chemist; enjoyed regular contact with Thomas Hariot, who filled the role of his steward; and served his term alongside other elite prisoners who shared his interest in distillation.[10]

Amazingly, an early recipe labeled "Our Great Cordiall" survives among Ralegh's papers, in his own hand no less.[11] The manuscript's jottings, however, offer only an abbreviated list of ingredients, suggesting that it is a work in progress, or perhaps even a false start; in fact, each line, except for the title and the first line, is crossed out individually:

> The tinctures drawne in spirit of wine of bur=
> rage floures,
> marigold floures
> red gillefloures
> rosa solis, of Cardus.
> of Angelica, of balme
> of margeram floures,
> of mint of settwell, of cardimomum of lignum aloes & of roses.
> Kermis, of Cubebs, of the tincture of Correl & gold.
> Cardimon.
> The whole bodies
> of ye magisterum of pearle,
> of unicorn, of amber greece, of muske,
> of terra silesiae, terra Ste pauli, terra sigillata of Turkie & florence.[12]

M. P. Earles suggests that Ralegh's surviving manuscript is a working copy, and that a scribe crossed out each ingredient while writing out a more complete version, one that he links to a British Library manuscript.[13] Nonetheless,

10 *Diary of the Rev. John Ward*, 168–69 as quoted in Nicholl, *The Creature in the Map*, 280, as well as Shirley, "The Scientific Experiments of Sir Walter Ralegh."

11 For a list of manuscripts that contain Ralegh's medical recipes, see Peter Beal, "Sir Walter Ralegh (1554–1618)," *Catalogue of English Literary Manuscripts 1450–1700*. Beal does not include the Sandys manuscript discussed here.

12 Walter Raleigh, *Chemical Recipes*, late sixteenth century–early seventeenth century, Sloane MS 359, British Library, London, England, 47v. My transcription is derived from a facsimile image of the manuscript recipe in M. P. Earles, "Our Great Cordiall," *Pharmaceutical Historian* 23, no. 1 (1983): 10.

13 Earles, "Our Great Cordiall," 10. See Raleigh, *Chemical Recipes*, late sixteenth century–early seventeenth century, Sloane MS 359, 47v.

the Ralegh manuscript's omission of ingredients that require importation from America is striking, given the scholarly drive to link the Great Cordial with Ralegh's transatlantic travels. This recipe specifies medicinal earths originally associated with European points of origin—the central European regions of Silesia, Malta, Turkey, and Florence[14]—and sea voyages were no doubt entwined in the need for pearl, coral, and ambergris. But nothing explicitly American is required in this concoction to link it to Guiana.

After his death, Ralegh's reputation for medicinal expertise grew, and stories of his learning and of the Great Cordial's origins combined to emphasize the importance of his voyages across the Atlantic. John Aubrey declared "Sir Walter Raleigh was a great chymist" and noted that he "studyed most in his Sea-Voyages, where he carried always a Trunke of Bookes along with him, and had nothing to divert him."[15] His name later appears on the list of "Persons of Quality" who "approved" through "Experience" the recipes published in the printed collection *Natura Exenterata* in 1655.[16] But these celebrations of Ralegh's experience offer little insight into what, if any, impact his travels had on his knowledge of medicines.

Among the early examples of the Great Cordial in a recipe manuscript, however, is one that casts doubt on how meaningful Ralegh's name is to the cure's survival. That is because his name is completely absent from the cure, and it is linked instead to a woman identified through the title Lady Sandys. The manuscript, held at the Princeton University Firestone Library and addressed in chapter 2, was started in the early seventeenth century and associated with the Sandys family—perhaps with Katherine Bulkeley Sandys (d. 1634), wife of Sir Edwin Sandys (1561–1629).[17] If this is indeed the correct Lady Sandys, this attribution would date the manuscript's Great Cordial recipe before 1634, the date of Katherine Sandys's death. An investor in the Virginia Company and its treasurer for one tumultuous year in 1619, Edwin Sandys and his family never traveled to Jamestown, but he

14 Dannenfeldt offers a helpful discussion of these often imprecise labels for medicinal earths in Karl H. Dannenfeldt, "The Introduction of a New Sixteenth-Century Drug," *Medical History* 28 (1984): 175.

15 John Aubrey, *Aubrey's Brief Lives* (Ann Arbor: University of Michigan Press, 1957), 254. Nicholl reinforces this connection, and Duckert remarks that "it is amusing to imagine Ralegh brushing up on his alchemy during the long voyage of 1595." See Nicholl, *The Creature in the Map*, 278 and Lowell Duckert, "Walter Ralegh's Liquid Narrative: *The Discoverie of Guiana*," in *Literary and Visual Ralegh*, ed. Christopher Armitage (Manchester: Manchester University Press, 2013), 234–25 for consideration of Ralegh's reading of alchemy on ship.

16 Philiatros, *Natura Exenterata: or Nature Unbowelled* (London: 1655), A r.

17 Theodore K. Rabb, "'My Lady Sandys her Receipts': A Manuscript of Cookery and Medicine," *The Princeton University Library Chronicle* 72, no. 2 (1969): 454–63.

was in constant contact with its governors about the colony's business.[18] Katherine, sickly for years after a harrowing labor and the subsequent stillbirth of her son,[19] certainly never ventured to the Americas, and her health kept her husband from venturing far from their English home. Recipes associated with the manuscript nonetheless show an enthusiasm for American ingredients and imported materials more broadly, perhaps for commercial reasons.

The Sandys version of the Great Cordial differs greatly from the one in Ralegh's manuscript, in that it illustrates the extent to which the cure combines ingredients from English fields with those imported from England's developing colonies. The compiler announces after roughly fifty pages of recipes, "Hear begins my Lady | Sandys her receipts."[20] The first full recipe, for "The great Cordiall," calls for three dozen ingredients, but only one—"Sassafras of Verginia" —is required to come from a specific, named geographical source:

> The great Cordiall
> Take borage flowers, rosemary flowers
> marygold flowers, red gilleflowers, rose-
> a solis, elder flowers, or each one pottle
> after they be dryed in the shade; alse
> of Scordium, cardus, angelica, balme,
> mint, margerome, Settwalle, betony, of
> each four handfulls, after they are dryed
> in the shade, of the rinds of Sassafras of
> Verginea, lignum aloes, of each four ounces
> beaten to pouder, of kermes, cubabes, car=
> damum, seduary, of each one ounce,
> of saffron halfe an ounce, Juniper berries
> tormetill roots, round bierwort roots,

18 Theodore K. Rabb, "Sandys, Sir Edwin (1561–1629), Politician and Colonial Entrepreneur," in *Oxford Dictionary of National Biography*, September 23, 2004, accessed July 18, 2023.

19 Rabb, "Sandys, Sir Edwin (1561–1629)."

20 *English Receipt Book*, seventeenth century, Princeton MS RTC01 No. 208, Princeton University, Princeton, NJ, 27v. After the announcement of Lady Sandys's section, the next text is large and centered, suggesting it should be read as a recipe header: "The Cordiall for convultione | fitts either in children or old folks | or for weaknesse." This could certainly be the title for a recipe that was never copied, or it could be a listing of the uses for the recipe that follows and which is identified on the next line as "The great Cordiall." See *English Receipt Book*, seventeenth century, Princeton MS RTC01 No. 208, 28r. The Great Cordial was often used to treat convulsions, as Rabb suggests. See Rabb, "My Lady Sandys her Receipts," 457.

> of each one ounce, or gentian roots halfe
> an ounce.
>
> Draw the tincture or extract of these
> with spirit of wine in balneo and save all
> the ingredients, after you have taken out
> the tincture and burnt them, and put their
> salts to their tinctures
>
> Take six ounce of the extracted of all
> these, with their salts, and put them the
> tincture of corrall three ounces, terra sigillata
> four drams, pearle prepared two ounces,
> Beasour stone three drammes, harts horne
> calcined four drames, ambergrees four drams,
> muske thirty graines, sugar candy one pound
> and a halfe, you must grinde your sugar very
> small and searce it through a fine searser,
> then the muske and amber must be ground and
> by little and little put amongst it, for the
> more you grinde the amber the better, then
> just so the sugar candy and all other dry
> materialls before directed, and make all
> as small as possible can be, then upon a great
> hollow painters grinding stone, mingle
> the tincturs and dry things togeather, which
> must be done by a stronge man, used to that
> labour, and while it is grinding put of red
> rose water syrrop of lemmons, and syrrup of
> red roses, equall quantities into it for else it
> will be so dry that it will not grinde or
> mingle to it, and commixt as it should be.[21]

Sassafras—and not just any sassafras, but Virginia sassafras—mingles here with native English flowers, ones that Lady Sandys could easily find on the family's Yorkshire estate, or in the fields around London or in its apothecary shops. But other ingredients are less common. Though it is mixed in with English plants like marjoram and betony, the tuberous plant

21 *English Receipt Book*, seventeenth century, Princeton MS RTC01 No. 208, 28r–29r.

setwall, or zedoary, would have been imported from the East Indies, as would have cubebs, berries of a shrub found in Java.[22] Similarly, the red insects known as *kermes* would have been imported from northern Africa or an intermediary port in southern Europe.[23] The medicinal earth, terra sigillata, would likely have been imported, as would the ambergris. Blending these ingredients from both East and West with spices like cardamom and saffron—which had long been imported to England, but which were nonetheless expensive[24]—the recipe exemplifies the global possibilities envisioned in seventeenth-century domestic recipes.

The same recipe—under the title "S[i]r Walter Rawleighs great Cordiall after | S[i]r Robert Killegrew's Way" —appears in a late seventeenth-century recipe manuscript, Wellcome Library MS 1340, associated with the Boyle family.[25] The manuscript has been credited to Katherine Jones, Lady Ranelagh (1615–91), and, more recently, to her sister-in-law, Margaret Boyle, Countess of Orrery (1623–89). As Michelle DiMeo stresses, though, this drive to establish a single author of the manuscript "simplifies the multiple layers of knowledge from several decades, evidenced in this manuscript."[26] Associating the recipe with a single family member becomes even more challenging upon noting the appearance of the recipe in Robert Boyle's printed *Some Considerations Touching the Vsefulnesse of Experimental Naturall Philosophy* in 1663.[27] Appearing under the heading "*S*[i]*r Walter Rawleighs* Cordial, after *S*[i]*r R. K.* his way: (set down *Verbatim* as I received it.)," Boyle's printed version is virtually identical to that in the family recipe book, though the handwriting in that manuscript is not his.[28] The family ties grow even stronger given that Boyle invokes the recipe in a section of *Some Considerations* that directly addresses his sister Lady Ranelagh's son Richard Jones, under the moniker Pyrophilus. Boyle reminds Pyrophilus of

22 See "setwall, n.," in *Oxford English Dictionary*, accessed September 23, 2023; "East India Company," "Ear–Easy chair," in Nancy Cox and Karin Dannehl, eds., Dictionary of Traded Goods and Commodities 1550–1820 (Wolverhampton: University of Wolverhampton, 2007), *British History Online*, accessed September 17, 2019.

23 "kermes, n.," in *Oxford English Dictionary*, accessed July 18, 2023.

24 See Paul Freedman, *Out of the East: Spices and the Medieval Imagination* (New Haven: Yale University Press, 2008), especially chapter 4.

25 Boyle Family, *Collection of 712 Medical Receipts*, 1675, Wellcome MS 1340, Wellcome Collection, London, England, 43v–44r.

26 Michelle DiMeo, "Lady Ranelagh's Book of Kitchen-Physick?: Reattributing Authorship for Wellcome Library MS 1340," *Huntington Library Quarterly* 77, no. 3 (2014): 343.

27 Boyle, *Some Considerations*, 316–17.

28 DiMeo offers an extensive analysis of the manuscript hands in DiMeo, "Lady Ranelagh's Book of Kitchen-Physick?"

an occasion when a suffering man was cured by "a large Dosis of Sir *Walter Rawleigh's* Cordial, sent him by an excellent Lady you are nearly related to."[29] Whether this is Lady Ranelagh or another relative, the comment returns the Great Cordial back to the Boyle's domestic realm, where it is administered by a woman of the household who may well have distilled it.

Not only is it unclear who in the Boyle family received the recipe, its title suggests that the recipe, with its Virginia sassafras, arrived after traveling through at least two sets of hands: Sir Walter Ralegh's and Sir Robert Killigrew's.[30] Killigrew, though not now a household name, carried a great deal of economic and social clout at the time, and he may have served as a link between Ralegh and the Sandys family. Killigrew helped Edwin Sandys secure a seat in Parliament early in his career,[31] and Killigrew was friendly enough with Ralegh to visit him in prison in the Tower of London during his imprisonment, perhaps putting him in proximity of the distilling experiments that led to the Great Cordial.[32] In addition, Killigrew's daughter Elizabeth married one of the Boyle siblings, Francis 1st Viscount of Shannon in 1638 or 39, opening up another line of communication that could have landed the recipe in the Boyle family hands.[33] These connections echo the complicated and obscure routes we have seen in other recipes taken from manuscript to manuscript.

In later pages of his work, Boyle claims a more direct access to an authoritative manuscript copy, underscoring exactly how quickly such recipes vacillate between the private and the public realm. He adopts an apologetic standpoint initially, arguing that he is "induc'd" to publish the recipe to assure its accuracy, perhaps as a corrective to Le Fèbure's demonstration and published discussion of the cordial's ingredients. Boyle further asserts that his version "has been abundantly recommended by Experience" unlike those that "pretended to be the true."[34] That probatum

29 Boyle, *Some Considerations*, 123.

30 The Boyle family actually bought their home, Lismore Castle, from Ralegh in 1602, though that need not suggest any direct recipe access. See Michelle DiMeo, *Lady Ranelagh: The Incomparable Life of Robert Boyle's Sister* (Chicago: University of Chicago Press, 2021), 18.

31 Alastair Bellany, "Killigrew, Sir Robert (1579/80–1633), courtier," in Oxford *Dictionary of National Biography*, September 23, 2004, accessed October 25, 2024.

32 Anne Duffin and Paul Hunneyball, "KILLIGREW, Sir Robert (c.1580–1633), of Kempton Park, Mdx.; Lothbury, London and Pendennis Castle, Cornw.," in *The History of Parliament: The House of Commons 1604–1629*, eds. Andrew Thrush and John P. Ferris (Cambridge: Cambridge University Press, 2010).

33 DiMeo, "Appendix: Boyle Family Genealogy," in *Lady Ranelagh*. Elizabeth was also King Charles II's mistress. See Bellany, "Killigrew, Sir Robert (1579/80–1633), courtier."

34 Boyle, *Some Considerations*, 316–17.

sets his version, which he claims is not just Killigrew's version but Ralegh's own, in opposition to others that circulated at the time. Access to the source, he implies, eliminates the interference imposed by other versions of the recipe; he claims the version he ushers into print maintains a direct link to its originator, which testifies to its purity. Boyle's urge to return to Ralegh's version situates the adjustments made in subsequent versions of the recipe as misguided tinkering, even corruptions, of an established formula, rather than improvements or modifications for an individual's needs. There is, he states, a "true" version, one that needs to be restored to prominence. Conveniently, the "true" version—the one linked to Ralegh—also proved effective in Boyle's own "Experience," aligning the authority of the recipe's attribution with that of its real-life implementation.

But here it must be said that the version Boyle publishes, and the virtually identical recipe in the Boyle family manuscript, offer only slight variations from the directions set down among Lady Sandys's receipts. True, the Sandys manuscript does not invoke Ralegh or any other intermediary, instead stressing in its header the medical uses the Great Cordial serves. Yet the versions' ingredients and proportions are identical, and they maintain much of the same idiosyncratic language of instruction.[35] And in offering guidance in making the tincture of coral required for the Cordial, all three offer a sketchy drawing—even the printed version—of a "long Glass with a narrow mouth" with another glass put "into the Mouth of it (the belly | upwards to save the vinegar from wasting)" (figures 5, 6, and 7).[36]

Though different versions of the Great Cordial recipe show a clear relationship to one another, they also underscore the inscrutable nature of the paths recipes travel. These manuscripts involve the names of well-documented families, and they contain copies of a recipe associated with the legendary Sir Walter Ralegh. But these connections ultimately lend little certainty to

35 For example, the Sandys manuscript insists that the maker "upon a great | hollow painters grinding stone, mingle | the tincturs and dry things togeather, which | must be done by a stronge man," while the Boyle family manuscript asks that "upon a great hollow grinding | stone mingle the tinctures and dry Ingredients together which must | be done by a Strong Man used to that Labour." Boyle's printed version contains only slight variations, telling the maker to "upon a great hallow grinding Stone mingle the Tinctures, and dry things together: (which must be done by a strong man used to that work)." *English Receipt Book*, seventeenth century, Princeton MS RTC01 No. 208, 28v–29r; Boyle Family, *Collection of 712 Medical Receipts*, 1675, Wellcome MS 1340, 43v–44r; Boyle, *Some Considerations*, 318.

36 This verbiage is exactly the same in all three versions, though the punctuation and capitalization vary. The quoted version is from the Boyle Family, *Collection of 712 Medical Receipts*, 1675, Wellcome MS 1340, 44r; see also Boyle, *Some Considerations*, 316 and the Sandys *English Receipt Book*, seventeenth century, Princeton MS RTC01 No. 208, 29r.

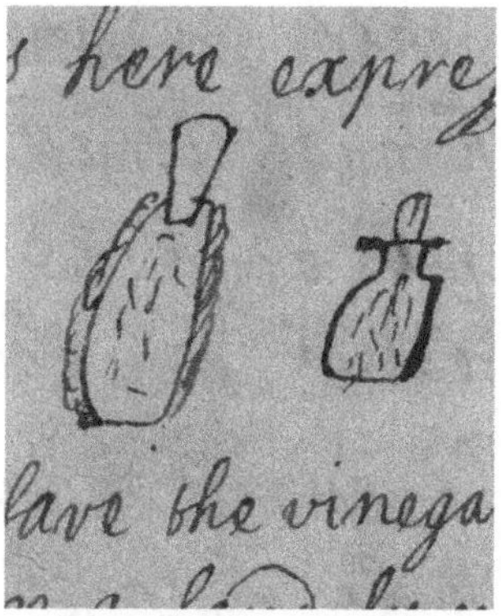

Figure 5. Illustration accompanying instructions for making the coral tincture used in the "Great Cordial" recipe in the Sandys Family Recipe Book, *English Receipt Book*, seventeenth century, Princeton MS RTC01 no. 208, Princeton University, 29r; Courtesy of Manuscripts Division, Department of Special Collections, Princeton University Library.

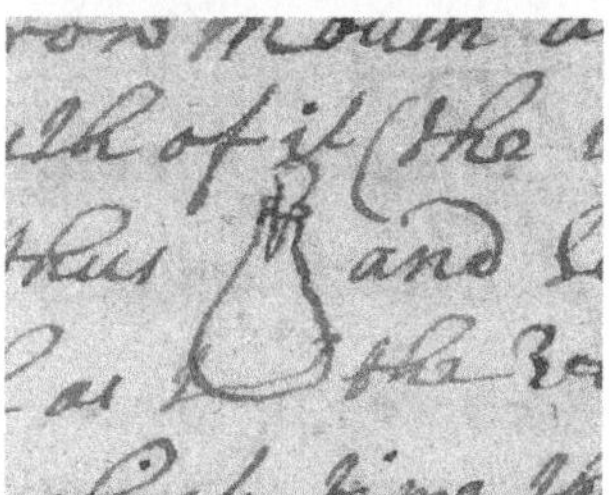

Figure 6. Illustration accompanying instructions for making the coral tincture used in the "Great Cordial" recipe in the Boyle family's *Collection of 712 Medical Receipts*, 1675, Wellcome MS 1340, 44r. Courtesy of the Wellcome Collection.

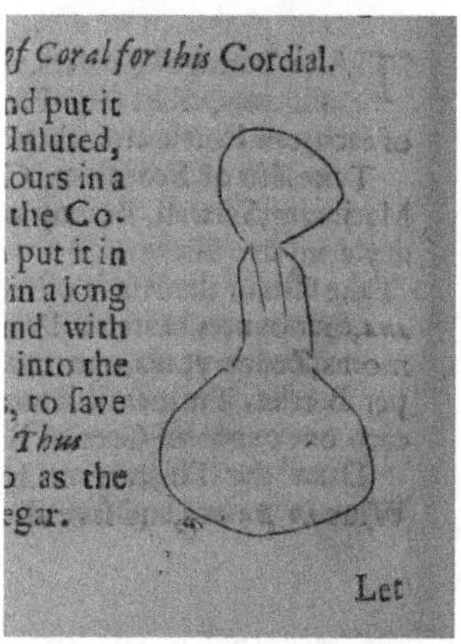

Figure 7. Illustration accompanying instructions for making the coral tincture used in the "Great Cordial" recipe in the Boyle's *Some Considerations Touching the Usefulnesse of Experimental Naturall Philosophy*, 1663, 318. Courtesy of the Wellcome Collection.

the recipe's history. Perhaps the Sandys version reflects access to the recipe as preserved by Ralegh's son, something that their Virginia connections may well have facilitated. Or the Sandys manuscript may suggest that Lady Sandys enjoyed a link to the Boyle household; since Katherine Sandys died in 1634, this might require rethinking which Lady Sandys the recipe book refers to. The endurance of the requirement for Virginia sassafras strengthens the bond between the two versions, but it offers no concrete explanations. Other versions of the Great Cordial recipe in manuscript, in fact, insist on those Virginia origins as well even as they introduce elements that further confuse attribution and accuracy. The compiler of a section of Sloane MS 359 labels a copy of the Great Cordial, and a group of other recipes, as "transcribed out of Sr Walter Raleghs booke of receipts written w[i]th his owne hand and is done according to the originall in everie sillable"; its Great Cordial recipe requiring *Sarzephras virginiae* as well.[37] In 1682, on the other hand, George Hartman's printed *The True Preserver and Restorer of Health* features a reformatted version of the recipe, calling it "Sir *Walter Releigh's* great Cordial according to the Counsel and Advice of Sir *Ken. Digby* and Sir *Alexander Fraiser*," with virtually identical ingredients. Maintaining its call for "Sassafras of Virginia," the recipe nonetheless eliminates Killigrew and adds Digby, a recognized courtier and Royal Society member,[38] and Frasier, a member of the College of Physicians.[39]

Moving with the Times

Perhaps ironically, this Great Cordial appears in no early American recipe books I have seen, in print or in manuscript. American recipe collections often included cordials, as the repeated appearances of Dr. Steven's Water make clear, and many other favored cures that called for the use of stills, but this recipe might have proven too complicated for colonial production. Perhaps the Great Cordial recipe itself does not cross oceans well, even as it relies on its ingredients doing so. In that sense, it repeats the explorer's methods of gathering materials from around the world, distilling the riches of empire for those living in England's abundance.

Yet the recipe nonetheless underscores the dangers of travel for those who leave England, at least as Le Fèbure interprets it. In explaining the uses of the Great Cordial, Le Fèbure returns to the *Airs, Waters, Places* tradition, implying that geography is destiny when it comes to bodily health. The Great Cordial, he asserts, "is wholly necessary for the Northerly and Sea-bordering people, and specially for the Inhabitants of Islands, by reason that all its Ingredients are filled with a concentred Light, which can remedy all their

37 See Raleigh, *Chemical Recipes*, late sixteenth century–early seventeenth century, Sloane MS 359, 47v.

38 Michael Foster, "Digby, Sir Kenelm (1603–1665), natural philosopher and courtier," in *Oxford Dictionary of National Biography*, September 23, 2004, accessed October 25, 2023.

39 Margaret Pelling and Frances White, "FRASER, Sir Alexander," in *Physicians and Irregular Medical Practitioners in London 1550–1640 Database* (London: Centre for Metropolitan History, 2004).

evils." Even as he calls on the alchemical notion of light as spirit, Le Fèbure repeats the long-established Hippocratic idea that island-dwellers, like the northerly English, suffer specific diseases because of their surroundings:

> In the first place, as concerning the Air and the Winds that reign with a perpetual inconstancy, all those that live in those Countries know too well by their own experience, that the Fogs and the humid Vapours of the Morning, as also those in the Evening … do so alter the Head and Breast, that one can scarcely be cautious enough, in whatsoever season it be, to prevent Defluxions and Rheums, Catarrhs, troublesome Coughs and Colds, which commonly draw after them Rheumatisms, wandering pains, Asthma's, the Lungs disease and the Consumption.[40]

Thus, even as the Great Cordial recipe embodies the urge to move beyond the land of one's birth, and in fact calls on the idealized romance of travel for its roots, it underscores the challenges such travel brings. At the same time, Le Fèbure's explanation acknowledges a link between English bodies and those the country's natives encounter when abroad. How else could American ingredients be effective against the conditions suffered by the English? Notably, Le Fèbure describes the English as vulnerable to the conditions that foreground "rheumatisms," a collection of symptoms whose title had only entered the wider English vocabulary after American exploration took hold. Such new perceptions of existing conditions required new treatments, ideally taken from lands that first spawned them. No wonder Virginia's sassafras remained key to the Great Cordial's composition.

The Great Cordial illustrates that recipes in domestic manuscripts have a public life, moving through society even as they concentrate on household health. These manuscripts acknowledge that individuals may leave home, severing their immediate bond to a place, but that connections to these locales endure, continuing to influence, if not govern, a traveler's health—that is, at least according to the *Airs, Waters, Places* tradition. The waters and botanical ingredients used to create medical cures mattered, because those ingredients carried with them the qualities of the lands that produced them. Those qualities, moreover, brought about unique reactions within the individual suffering body, and those reactions were determined in part by the geographical conditions of the patient's birth. Even at a time when journeying across the Atlantic to make new permanent settlements there became possible, these Hippocratic notions of bodily ties

40 Le Fèbure, *A Discourse upon Sr Walter Rawleigh's Great Cordial*, 97–98.

to homelands remained embedded in English medical recipes as produced and used in the home, suggesting both a sense of nostalgia and a fear of severing ancestral ties.

The same recipes that embodied these notions of home—reflected in their easy assumptions of access to ingredients, whether freshly gathered from nearby fields or purchased from local markets—traveled to places where such access would prove challenging, if not impossible, even though goods moved with increasing ease through the Atlantic world. As recipes made their way into London from the countryside, and as they moved from England to the colonies, their origins became increasingly obscured. Pinning down where a cure was first made is rarely possible, even when the names associated with a medical preparation, and the ingredients in it, offer tempting clues to its roots. To look for these roots, after all, is to take the principles of *Airs, Waters, Places* seriously, as a lived rule for best practices in medical care. The fact that recipes routinely set aside those principles, mixing together the local and the imported, highlights the extent to which early modern English people were willing to make room for innovation in their home medical practice. Traditional methods need not be abandoned, just as a grandmother's cures could be retained in a manuscript even if never used. New cures, for newly recognized conditions as well as pernicious old ones, could simply be added, appended to the inherited record. In that sense, early modern recipe manuscripts record travel even when they do not move substantially in their own right. They instead absorb the movements of ingredients, whole recipes, and individual practitioners, recording the new ideas and experiences influencing medical thinking in the domestic realm. As homebound as they may seem to be, these manuscripts highlight the permeable borders of the seemingly clearly demarcated domestic realm, demonstrating the home medical recipes moved with the times, and with the people who valued the knowledge conveyed through their pages.

A Note on Conventions

Transcriptions of early modern recipe manuscripts and print texts are increasingly available digitally, and this book incorporates these sources when they are freely accessible. When available and searchable via the Folger Shakespeare Library online catalog, I have used provided transcriptions of early modern recipe books to increase accessibility, noting any changes in brackets on the rare occasions where intervention is required. Otherwise, all manuscript transcriptions are my own unless specifically noted, and they embody the principles of semi-diplomatic transcription, silently lowering superscripts and expanding common abbreviations. Similarly, I have used transcriptions created by the Early English Books Online Text Creation Partnership when citing printed texts that appear in the Early English Books Online collection. These practices account for some variations in the rendering of *u* and *v* in quoted texts.

Bibliography

Alaimo, Stacy. *Bodily Natures: Science, Environment, and the Material Self.* Bloomington and Indianapolis: University of Indiana Press, 2010.

Albala, Ken. "Stimulants and Intoxicants in Europe, 1500–1700." In *The Routledge History of Food,* edited by C. Helstosky, 42–60. London: Routledge, 2014.

Allen, Katherine. "Newspaper Remedies and Commercial Medicine in Eighteenth-Century Recipe Books." *The Recipes Project,* January 4, 2014. Accessed October 14, 2024. https://recipes.hypotheses.org/3584.

Allen, Katherine. "Recipe Collections and the Realities of Fashionable Diseases in Eighteenth-Century Elite Domestic Medicine." *Literature and Medicine* 35, no. 2 (2017): 334–54.

"America and West Indies: January 1623." In *Calendar of State Papers, Colonial, America and West Indies: Volume 1: 1574–1660,* edited by W. Noel Sainsbury, 35–37. London, 1860. *British History Online.* Accessed October 14, 2024. https://www.british-history.ac.uk/cal-state-papers/colonial/america-west-indies/vol1/pp35-37.

"ammoniac, adj. & n." *Oxford English Dictionary.* Accessed June 18, 2022, https://doi.org/10.1093/OED/1097328460.

Appelbaum, Robert. "Hunger in Early Virginia: Indians and English Facing Off over Excess, Want, and Need." In *Envisioning an English Empire: Jamestown and the Making of the North Atlantic World,* edited by Robert Appelbaum and John Wood Sweet, 195–216. Philadelphia: University of Pennsylvania Press, 2005.

Archer, Jayne Elisabeth. "'An Offering to her Memory': Healing, Motherhood, and Identity in the Manuscript Remains of Lady Ann Fanshawe." In *Identities in Early Modern English Writing: Religion, Gender, Nation,* edited by Lorna Fitzsimmons, 117–43. Vol. 6 of *Early European Research.* Turnhout: Brepols, 2014.

Ashton, Robert. "Revenue Farming under the Early Stuarts." *Economic History Review* 8, no. 3 (1956): 310–22.

Aubrey, John. *Aubrey's Brief Lives.* Ann Arbor: University of Michigan Press, 1957.

Ayscough, Lady. *Receits of Phisick and Chirurgery.* 1692. Wellcome MS 1026. Wellcome Collection, London, England.

Bacon, Catherine. *Receipt Book of Catherine Bacon.* ca. 1680–1739. Folger MS V.a.621. Folger Shakespeare Library, Washington, DC.

Balleine, G. R. *All for the King: The Life Story of Sir George Carteret.* St. Helier, Jersey: Société Jersiaise, 1976.

Barrett, Lady. *Select Receipts.* 1711. Wellcome MS 1071. Wellcome Collection, London, England.

Bashford, Alison and Sarah W. Tracy. "Introduction: Modern Airs, Waters, and Places." *Bulletin of the History of Medicine* 86, no. 4 (2012): 495–514.

Bassnett, Madeline. "A Language Not One's Own: Translational Exchange in Seventeenth-Century Englishwomen's Iberian Recipes." *Journal of Early Modern Cultural Studies* 19, no. 1 (2019): 1–27.

Bassnett, Madeline. *Women, Food Exchange, and Governance in Early Modern England.* New York: Palgrave Macmillan, 2016.

Batman, Stephen. *Batman uppon Bartholome.* London, 1582.

Baumfylde, Mary. *Medicinal and Cookery Recipes of Mary Baumfylde.* 1626. Folger MS V.a. 456. Folger Shakespeare Library, Washington, DC.

Beal, Peter. "Sir Walter Ralegh (1554–1618)." *Catalogue of English Literary Manuscripts 1450–1700.* Accessed October 14, 2024. https://celm.folger.edu/authors/raleghsirwalter.html.

Beecher, Donald. "John Frampton of Bristol: Trader and Translator." In *Travel and Translation in the Early Modern Period*, edited by Carmine G. Di Biase, 103–21. Amsterdam: Rodopi, 2006.

Beecher, Donald. "Nicolás Monardes, John Frampton and the Medical Wonders of the New World." In *Humanismo e ciência: Antiguidade erenascimento*, edited by António Manuel Lopes Andrade, Carlos de Miguel Mora, and João Manuel Nunes Torrão, 141–60. Coimbra: Imprensa da Universidade de Coimbra, 2015.

Belknap, Jeremy. *The History of New-Hampshire*. Boston: Belknap and Young, 1792.

Bell, Whitfield J., ed. "Nicholas Collin's Appeal to American Scientists." *William and Mary Quarterly* 13, no. 4 (1956): 519–50.

Bellany, Alastair. "Killigrew, Sir Robert (1579/80–1633), courtier." *Oxford Dictionary of National Biography*. September 23, 2004. Accessed October 25, 2024. doi-org.ezproxy.uakron.edu:2443/10.1093/ref:odnb/15537.

Benedek, Thomas G. *Rheumatism: Its History from the Advent of Experimental Science to the Impact of Bacteriology*. New York: Nova Biomedical, 2017.

Benedek, Thomas G. *Rheumatism: Its History from Paleo-Pathology to the Advent of Experimental Science*. New York: Nova Biomedical, 2015.

Benson, Evelyn Abraham. *Penn Family Recipes: Cooking Recipes of William Penn's Wife, Gulielma*. York, PA: George Shumway, 1966.

Bernhard, Virginia. "Men, Women and Children at Jamestown: Population and Gender in Early Virginia, 1607–1610." *Journal of Southern History* 58, no. 4 (1992): 599–618.

Best, Henry. *Rural Economy in Yorkshire in 1641, being the Farm and Account Books of Henry Best*, edited by Charles Best Robinson. Durham: Publications of the Surtees Society, 1857.

Beverley, Robert. *The History and Present State of Virginia: A New Edition with an Introduction by Susan Scott Parrish*, edited by Susan Scott Parrish. Chapel Hill: University of North Carolina Press, 2013. Accessed October 14, 2024. ProQuest Ebook Central.

Blakley, Christopher M. "'I have been obliged to Send Nassaw': An Enslaved Healer's Medical Labour and Skill in Eighteenth-Century Virginia." *Medical History* 65, no. 2 (2021): 121–39.

Blanton, Wyndham Bolling. *Medicine in Virginia in the Seventeenth Century*. New York: Arno Press, 1972.

Bleichmar, Daniela. "Books, Bodies, and Fields: Sixteenth-Century Transatlantic Encounters with New World *Materia Medica*." In *Colonial Botany: Science, Commerce, and Politics*, edited by Londa Schiebinger and Claudia Swan, 83–99. Philadelphia: University of Pennsylvania Press, 2005.

"'bole Armoniac' in ammoniac, adj., sense 1.b." *Oxford English Dictionary*. Accessed July 18, 2023, https://doi.org/10.1093/OED/1206713059.

Book of Receipts. 1731. Virginia Tech Ms 2008-024. Virginia Tech University, Blacksburg, VA.

A Book of Receipts, which was Given me by Several Men for Several Causes, Griefs and Diseases. ca. 1625–c. 1700. Folger MS V.a.361. Folger Shakespeare Library, Washington, DC.

A Booke of Sweetmeats. Eighteenth Century. *Historical Society of Pennsylvania Collection of George Washington Family Papers*. Historical Society of Pennsylvania, Philadelphia, PA.

Boyle Family. *Collection of 712 Medical Receipts*. 1675. Wellcome MS 1340. Wellcome Collection, London, England.

Boyle, Robert. *Some Considerations Touching the Vsefulnesse of Experimental Naturall Philosophy*. Oxford, 1663.

Brandt, Susan H. *Women Healers: Gender, Authority, and Medicine in Early Philadelphia*. Philadelphia: University of Pennsylvania Press, 2022.

Brigham, Charles. *Account Book [manuscript]*. 1650–1730s. American Antiquarian Society Mss. Folio Vols. B. American Antiquarian Society, Worcester, MA.

Bright, Timothie. *A Treatise, wherein is Declared the Sufficiencie of English Medicines*. London, 1615.

Brown, Alexander. *The First Republic in America*. Boston: Houghton, 1898.

Bruce, Philip Alexander. *Economic History of Virginia in the Seventeenth Century*. London: Macmillan, 1896.

Brumwich, Anne. *Mrs Anne Brumwich her Booke of Receipts or Medicines for Severall Sores and other Infermities*. 1625. Wellcome MS 160. Wellcome Collection, London, England.

Bullein, William. *The Government of Health*. London, 1595.

Burke, Victoria E. "Richardson [*née* Beaumont; *other married name* Ashburnham], Elizabeth, *suo jure* baroness of Cramond (1576/7–1651)." *Oxford Dictionary of National Biography*. January 3, 2008. Accessed October 31, 2024. doi-org.ezproxy.uakron.edu:2443/10.1093/ref:odnb/46468.

Butler, Matthew. "William Butler (1535–1618): A Biography of a Singular Physician." *Journal of Medical Biography* 1 (2023): 1–8.

Bye, Philip. "Ashburnham Recipe Book." Email message to author, June 20, 2018.

Cannon, John. "Carteret, John, second Earl Granville (1690–1763), politician." *Oxford Dictionary of National Biography*. September 23, 2004. Accessed August 25, 2023. doi-org.ezproxy.uakron.edu:2443/10.1093/ref:odnb/4804.

Carteret, Grace. *Manuscript Recipe Book of Grace Carteret, 1st Countess Granville*. 1654–1744. Welcome MS. 8903. Wellcome Collection, London, England.

Cartier, Jacques. "A Shorte and Briefe Narration of the Navigation Made by the Commandment of the King of France, to the Islands of Canada." In *The Third and Last Volume of the Voyages, Navigations, Traffiques, and Discoveries of the English Nation*, edited by Richard Hakluyt, 212–32. London, 1600.

Castleton, Lady Grace. *The Lady Grace Castleton's Booke of Receipts*. Seventeenth century. Folger MS V.a. 600. Folger Shakespeare Library, Washington, DC.

Catchmay, Lady Frances. *A Booke of Medicens*. Seventeenth century. Wellcome MS 184a. Wellcome Collection, London, England.

Cavendish, Margaret. *The Worlds Olio*. London, 1655.

Chamberlayne, Edward. *Angliæ Notitia, or The Present State of England Together with Divers Reflections upon the Antient State Thereof*. London, 1669.

Chantrell, Mary. *Book of Receipts*. 1690. Wellcome MS.1548. Wellcome Collection, London, England.

Chaplin, Joyce E. "Earthsickness: Circumnavigation and the Terrestrial Human Body, 1520–1800." *Bulletin of the History of Medicine* 86 (2012): 515–42.

Chaplin, Joyce E. *Subject Matter: Technology, the Body, and Science on the Anglo-American Frontier, 1500–1676*. Cambridge, MA: Harvard University Press, 2003.

Chastellux, Marquis de. *Travels in North America in the Years 1780, 1781, and 1782*. Vol. 2. Translated by Howard C. Rice, Jr. Chapel Hill: University of North Carolina Press, 1963.

Chesterfield, Philip Dormer. *The Letters of Philip Dormer Stanhope, 4th Earl of Chesterfield*, edited by Bonamy Dobrée. New York: AMS Press, 1932.

Cirket, A. F. and Bette Stitt. *English Wills, 1498–1526; Diana Astry's Recipe Book c. 1700*. London: Boydell & Brewer, 1957.

Clayton, John. *The Reverend John Clayton: A Parson with a Scientific Mind*, edited by Edmund Berkeley and Dorothy Smith Berkeley. Charlottesville: Virginia Historical Society, 1965.

Cliffe, J. T. *The Yorkshire Gentry from the Reformation to the Civil War*. London: Athlone Press, 1969.

Cogan, Thomas. *The Haven of Health*. London, 1636.

Collin, Nicholas. "An Essay on Those Inquiries in Natural Philosophy, which at Present are most Beneficial to the United State of North America." In "Nicholas Collin's Appeal to American Scientists," edited by Whitfield J. Bell. *William and Mary Quarterly* 13, no. 4 (1956): 519–50.

Collinson, Patrick. "Sandys, Edwin (1519?–1588), archbishop of York." *Oxford Dictionary of National Biography*. September 23, 2004. Accessed October 14, 2024. doi-org.ezproxy.uakron.edu:2443/10.1093/ref:odnb/24649.

Connor, Kimberley G. "Seeking Margaret Baker: Identifying the Author of Three Manuscript Receipt Books." *ABO: Interactive Journal for Women in the Arts, 1640–1830* 12, no. 1 (2022): 1–29.

Console, Renzo. "Pharmaceutical Use of Gold from Antiquity to the Seventeenth Century." In *A History of Geology in Medicine*, edited by C. Duffin, R. T. J. Moody and C. Gardner-Thorpe, 171–91. London: Geological Society of London, 2013.

Cook, Harold J. "Markets and Cultures: Medical Specifics and the Reconfiguration of the Body in Early Modern Europe." *Transactions of the Royal Historical Society* 21 (2011): 123–45.

Cookbook. ca. 1700. Virginia Museum of History & Culture MS 5:5 Un 3:4. Virginia Historical Society, Richmond, VA.

Cookbook. ca. 1720. Folger MS W.b.653. Folger Shakespeare Library, Washington, DC.

Cooke, Nathalie and Kathryn Harvey, eds. *The Johnson Family Treasury: A Collection of Household Recipes and Remedies, 1741–1848*. Oakville, ON: Rock's Mills Press, 2015.

Cookery and Medicinal Receipts. 1820. University of Minnesota MS Small QV C773 1820. Owen H. Wangensteen Historical Library of Biology and Medicine, Minneapolis, MN.

Copeman, W. S. C. *A Short History of Gout and the Rheumatic Diseases*. Berkeley: University of California Press, 1964.

Corlyon, Mrs. *A booke of such medicines as have been approved by the speciall practize of Mrs. Corlyon*. ca. 1606. Folger MS V.a. 388. Folger Shakespeare Library, Washington, DC.

Cox, Nancy and Karin Dannehl, eds. *Dictionary of Traded Goods and Commodities 1550–1820*. Wolverhampton: University of Wolverhampton, 2007. *British History Online*. Accessed September 17, 2019.

Crawford, Matthew James and Joseph M. Gabriel, eds. *Drugs on the Page: Pharmacopoeias and Healing Knowledge in the Early Modern Atlantic World*. Pittsburgh: University of Pittsburgh Press, 2019.

Cruso, Mary and Timothy Cruso. *Cookbook of Mary Cruso and Timothy Cruso*. 1689. Folger MS X.d.24. Folger Shakespeare Library, Washington, DC.

"Cure for the Rheumatism." *Hobart Town Gazette and Van Diemen's Land Advertiser* (Tas.: 1821–25): September 20, 1823: 2. Accessed June 28, 2024. http://nla.gov.au/nla.news-article1089969.

Dannenfeldt, Karl H. "The Introduction of a New Sixteenth-Century Drug." *Medical History* 28 (1984): 174–88.

Dawson, Thomas. *The Good Husvvifes Ievvell*. London, 1587.

Davidson, Peter. "Fanshawe [*née* Harrison], Ann, Lady Fanshawe, autobiographer." *Oxford Dictionary of National Biography*. Oxford: Oxford University Press, 2004. September 23, 2004. Accessed October 14, 2024. doi-org.ezproxy.uakron.edu:2443/10.1093/ref:odnb/9146.

Deetz, Kelley Fanto. *Bound to the Fire: How Virginia's Enslaved Cooks Helped Invent American Cuisine*. Lexington: University Press of Kentucky Press, 2017.

DiMarco, Vincent. *It Has Helped to Admiration: Eighteenth-Century Medical Cures from the Kitchen Book of Bridget Lane*. Bloomington, IN: iUniverse, 2010.

DiMeo, Michelle. "Authorship and Medical Networks: Reading Attributions in Early Modern Manuscript Recipe Books." In *Reading and Writing Recipe Books, 1550–1800*, edited by Michelle DiMeo and Sara Pennell, 25–46. Manchester: Manchester University Press, 2013.

DiMeo, Michelle. "Lady Ranelagh's Book of Kitchen-Physick?: Reattributing Authorship for Wellcome Library MS 1340." *Huntington Library Quarterly* 77, no. 3 (2014): 331–46.

DiMeo, Michelle. *Lady Ranelagh: The Incomparable Life of Robert Boyle's Sister*. Chicago: University of Chicago Press, 2021.

DiMeo, Michelle and Sara Pennell, eds. *Reading and Writing Recipe Books, 1500–1800*. Manchester: Manchester University Press, 2013.

Duckert, Lowell. *For All Waters: Finding Ourselves in Early Modern Wetscapes*. Minneapolis: University of Minnesota Press, 2017.

Duckert, Lowell. "Water Ralegh's Liquid Narrative: *The Discoverie of Guiana*." In *Literary and Visual Ralegh*, edited by Christopher Armitage, 217–41. Manchester: Manchester University Press, 2013.

Duffin, Anne and Paul Hunneyball. "KILLIGREW, Sir Robert (c.1580–1633), of Kempton Park, Mdx.; Lothbury, London and Pendennis Castle, Cornw." In *The History of Parliament: The House of Commons 1604–1629*, edited by Andrew Thrush and John P. Ferris. Cambridge: Cambridge University Press, 2010.

Dugan, Holly. *The Ephemeral History of Perfume: Scent and Sense in Early Modern England*. Baltimore: Johns Hopkins University Press, 2011.

Eamon, William. *Science and the Secrets of Nature*. Princeton: Princeton University Press, 1994.

Earle, Rebecca. *The Body of the Conquistador: Food, Race and the Colonial Experience in Spanish America, 1492–1700*. Cambridge: Cambridge University Press, 2012.

Earles, M. P. "Our Great Cordiall." *Pharmaceutical Historian* 23, no. 1 (1983): 310–12.

Early Modern Manuscripts Online. https://emmo.folger.edu. Accessed September 20, 2024.

Early Modern Recipes Online Collective. https://emroc.hypotheses.org. Accessed September 20, 2024.

Eden, Trudy. "Food, Assimilation, and the Malleability of the Human Body in Early Virginia." In *A Centre of Wonders: The Body in Early America*, edited by Janet Moore Lindman and Michele Lise Tarter, 29–42. Ithaca: Cornell University Press, 2001.

Eklund, Hilary. "Wetlands Reclamation and the Fate of the Local in Seventeenth Century England." In *Ground-Work: English Renaissance Literature and Soil Science*, edited by Hilary Eklund, 149–70. University Park: Penn State University Press, 2017.

Elyot, Thomas. *The Castel of Health*. London, 1539.

Elyot, Thomas. *The Dictionary of Syr Thomas Eliot Knight*. London, 1538.

English Household and Medicinal Book. 1800s. University of Iowa En 36. University of Iowa, Iowa City, IA. https://digital.lib.uiowa.edu/islandora/object/ui%3Acookbooks_13531_2_2.

English Medicinal and Cookery Late 16th–mid-17th century. 1540–1670. University of Minnesota Libraries WZ240 E58 1540. Owen H. Wangensteen Historical Library of Biology and Medicine, Minneapolis, MN.

English, Peter C. *Rheumatic Fever in America and Britain: A Biological, Epidemiological, and Medical History*. New Brunswick, NJ: Rutgers University Press, 1999.

English Receipt Book. Seventeenth century. Princeton MS RTC01 no. 208. Princeton University, Princeton, NJ.

Erskine, Lady Mary Jean. *The First Part of this Booke of Phisicke*. 1650–1700. University of Minnesota Libraries MS Oversize WZ225 F527 1650. Owen H. Wangensteen Historical Library of Biology and Medicine, Minneapolis, MN.

Estienne, Charles. *Maison Rustique or The Country Farme*. London, 1616.

Evelyn, John. *The Diary and Correspondence of John Evelyn, F.R.S.*, edited by William Bray. London, 1857.

Every Man his own Doctor: or, The Poor Planter's Physician. Williamsburg, 1736.

Ewen, Misha. *The Virginia Venture: American Colonization and English Society, 1580–1660*. Philadelphia: University of Pennsylvania Press, 2022.

Fairfax, Elizabeth. *Manuscript Book of Culinary and Medicinal Recipes in Several Hands*. 1694. GMU MS C0202. George Mason University, Fairfax, VA.

"The Famous American Receipt for the Rheumatism." *The Gentleman's Magazine.* June 1, 1766: 280.

"The Famous American Receipt for the Rheumatism." *London Magazine: or, Gentleman's Monthly Intelligencer.* June 1, 1766: 324.

"The Famous American Receipt for the Rheumatism." *Royal Magazine.* June 1, 1766: 300.

"The Famous American Receipt for the Rheumatism." *The Universal Magazine of Knowledge and Pleasure.* June 1, 1766: 329.

Fanshawe, Ann. *The Memoirs of Ann, Lady Fanshawe.* In *The Memoirs of Anne, Lady Halkett and Ann, Lady Fanshawe*, edited by John Loftis, 101–92. Oxford: Clarendon, 1979.

Fanshawe, Ann. *The Memoirs of Ann, Lady Fanshawe, Wife of Sir Richard Fanshawe, bart., 1600–72*, edited by Herbert Charles Fanshawe. London: J. Lane, 1907.

Fanshawe, Ann. *Mrs. Fanshawes Booke of Receipts of Physickes Salues, Waters, Cordials, Preserves and Cookery.* 1678. Wellcome MS 7113. Wellcome Library, London, England.

Fanshawe, H. C. *The History of the Fanshawe Family.* Newcastle upon Tyne: A. Reid, 1927.

Feerick, Jean. *Strangers in Blood: Relocating Race in the Renaissance.* Toronto: University of Toronto Press, 2010.

Fenton, William N. *Contacts between Iroquois Herbalism and Colonial Medicine.* Seattle: Shorey Book Store, 1971.

Field, Catherine. "'Many Hands Hands': Writing the Self in Early Modern Women's Recipe Books." In *Genre and Women's Life Writing in Early Modern England*, edited by Michelle M. Dowd and Julie Eckerle, 49–63. Aldershot: Ashgate, 2007.

Fine, Gary Alan and Patricia A Turner. *Whispers on the Color Line: Rumor and Race in America.* Berkeley: University of California Press, 2001.

Fissell, Mary E. "Women, Health, and Healing in Early Modern Europe." *Bulletin of the History of Medicine* 82, no. 1 (2008): 1–17.

Fitzhugh, Ellen. *Manuscript Recipe Book.* 1842. University of Pennsylvania Ms. Codex 651. University of Pennsylvania, Philadelphia, PA.

Fleming, Abraham. *A Memorial of the Famous Monuments and Charitable Almsdeedes of the Right Worshipfull Maister William Lambe.* London, 1580.

Floyd-Wilson, Mary. "English Mettle." In *Reading the Early Modern Passions: Essays in the Cultural History of Emotion*, edited by Gail Kern Paster, Katherine Rowe, and Mary Floyd-Wilson, 130–46. Philadelphia: University of Pennsylvania Press, 2004.

Fogarty, Ann. "Reading Dislocation and Emotion in the Writings of Alice Thornton, Ann Fanshawe, and Barbara Blaugdone." In *Women's Life Writing and Early Modern Ireland*, edited by Julie A. Eckerle and Naomi McAreavey, 51–76. Lincoln: University of Nebraska Press, 2019.

Foley, Christopher D. "Marlowe's *Edward II* and 'The Woful Lamentations of Jane Shore': Tactical Engagements with Sewers in Late-Elizabethan England." *Early Modern Literary Studies* 23 (2014). Accessed October 14, 2024. https://extra.shu.ac.uk/emls/journal/indexphp/emls/article/download/179/179-828-1-PB.pdf.

Foreman, Richard and Jas. W. Mahoney. *The Cherokee Physician, or Indian Guide to Health.* Chapel Hill: University of North Carolina at Chapel Hill Library, 2018.

Foster, Michael. "Digby, Sir Kenelm (1603–1665), Natural Philosopher and Courtier." *Oxford Dictionary of National Biography.* September 23, 2004. Accessed October 25, 2023. doi-org.ezproxy.uakron.edu:2443/10.1093/ref:odnb/7629.

"fountain-water, n." *Oxford English Dictionary.* Accessed September 23, 2023, https://doi.org/10.1093/OED/1099282238.

Foust, Clifford M. *Rhubarb: The Wondrous Drug.* Princeton: Princeton University Press, 1992.

Frankland, Lady. *Recipe Book.* 1750–1825. University of Pennsylvania Ms. Codex 644. University of Pennsylvania, Philadelphia, PA.

Freedman, Paul. *Out of the East: Spices and the Medieval Imagination*. New Haven: Yale University Press, 2008.

French, John. *The Art of Distillation*. London, 1651.

Gabriel, Joseph M. "Indian Secrets, Indian Cures, and the Pharmacopoeia of the United States of America." In *Drugs on the Page: Pharmacopoeias and Healing Knowledge in the Early Modern Atlantic World*, edited by Matthew James Crawford and Joseph M. Gabriel, 240–62. Pittsburgh: University of Pittsburgh Press, 2019.

Gallay, Alan. *Walter Ralegh: Architect of Empire*. New York: Basic, 2019.

Garrod, Alfred Baring. *The Nature and Treatment of Gout and Rheumatic Gout*. London, 1859.

Gerard, John. *The Herball or Generall History of Plantes*. London, 1633.

Goldstein, David B. *Eating and Ethics in Shakespeare's England*. Cambridge: Cambridge University Press, 2013.

Goldstein, David B. and Amy L. Tigner. *Culinary Shakespeare: Staging Food and Drink in Early Modern England*. Pittsburgh: Duquesne University Press, 2016.

Gómez, Pablo F. "[Un]Muffled Histories: Translating Bodily Practices in the Early Modern Caribbean." *Osiris* 37 (2022): 233–50.

Gordon, Sarah. "Mens Sana in Corpore Sanus: Water, Wellness, and Cleanliness in Five Fifteenth-Century Medical Manuals." In *Bodily and Spiritual Hygiene in Medieval and Early Modern Literature: Explorations of Textual Presentations of Filth and Water*, edited by Albrecht Classen, 434–40. Berlin: De Gruyter, 2017.

Granville Family. *Cookery and Medical Receipts of the Granville Family. c. 1640–c. 1750*. Folger MS V.a. 430. Folger Shakespeare Library, Washington, DC.

Griffin, Clare. "Disentangling Commodity Histories: Pauame and Sassafras in the Early Modern Global World." *Journal of Global History* 15, no. 1 (2020): 1–18.

Hall, Constance. *Receipt Book*. 1672. Folger MS V.a.20. Folger Shakespeare Library, Washington, DC.

Hall, David D. "The Chesapeake in the Seventeenth Century." In *A History of the Book in America: Vol. 1: The Colonial Book in the Atlantic World*, edited by Hugh Amory and David D. Hall, 55–82. Chapel Hill: University of North Carolina Press, 2007.

Hall, Kim F. "Culinary Spaces, Colonial Spaces: The Gendering of Sugar in the Seventeenth Century." In *Feminist Readings of Early Modern Culture: Emerging Subjects*, edited by Valerie Traub and M. Lindsay Kaplan, 168–90. Cambridge: University of Cambridge, 1996.

Harbury, Katherine E. *Colonial Virginia's Cooking Dynasty*. Columbia: University of South Carolina Press, 2004.

Hardin, William. "'Pipe-Pilgrimages' and 'Fruitfull Rivers': Thomas Middleton's Civic Entertainments and the Water Supply of Early Modern London." *Renaissance Papers* (1993): 63–74.

Hariot, Thomas. *A Briefe and True Report of the New Found Land of Virginia*. London, 1590.

Harris, Jonathan Gil. "This Is Not a Pipe: Water Supply Incontinent Sources, and the Leaky Body Politic." In *Enclosure Acts*, edited by Richard Burt, 203–28. Ithaca: Cornell University Press, 1994.

Harrison, Francis Burton. "Harrisons in Virginia during the Reign of James I (Concluded)." *The Virginia Magazine of History and Biography* 51, no. 4 (1943): 326–38.

Hart, James. *Klinike, or The Diet of the Diseased*. London, 1633.

Havard, Lucy J. "Preserve or Perish: Food Preservation Practices in the Early Modern Kitchen." *Notes and Records* 74 (2020): 5–33.

Hayes, Kevin J. *A Colonial Woman's Bookshelf*. Knoxville: University of Tennessee Press, 1996.

Healy, Simon. "CONSTABLE, Sir Henry (1556/7–1607), of Burton Constable and Upsall Castle, Yorks." In *The History of Parliament: The House of Commons 1604–1629*, edited by Andrew Thrush and John P. Ferris. Cambridge: Cambridge University Press, 2010. Accessed

October 14, 2024. https://www.historyofparliamentonline.org/volume/1604-1629/member/constable-sir-henry-15567-1607.

Healy, Simon. "HARRISON, John (c.1589–1669), of St. Olave's, Hart Street, London; later of Balls Park, Herts. and Beaumont, Lancs." *The History of Parliament: The House of Commons 1604–1629*, edited Andrew Thrush and John P. Ferris. Cambridge: Cambridge University Press, 2010. Accessed October 14, 2024. http://www.historyofparliamentonline.org/volume/1604–1629/member/harrison-john-1589-1669.

Heller, Jennifer. *The Mother's Legacy in Early Modern England*. Basingstoke: Ashgate, 2011.

Herbert, Amanda. *Female Alliances: Gender, Identity, and Friendship in Early Modern Britain*. New Haven: Yale University Press, 2014.

Hermann, Rachel. B. "The 'Tragicall Historie': Cannibalism and Abundance in Colonial Jamestown." *The William and Mary Quarterly* 68, no. 1 (2011): 47–74.

Hess, Karen, ed. *Martha Washington's Booke of Cookery*. New York: Columbia, 1981.

Hodgkin, Katherine. "Women, Memory and Family History in Seventeenth-Century England." In *Memory before Modernity: Practices of Memory in Early Modern Europe*, edited by Erika Kuijpers, Judith Pollmann, Johannes Müller, and Jasper van der Steen, 297–313. Leiden: Brill, 2013.

Holloway, Anne and Ramona Wray. "'O daughter ... forget your people and your father's house': Early Modern Women Writers and the Spanish Imaginary." *Bulletin of Spanish Studies* 9 (2016): 1387–413.

Hyde, Bridget. *Madam Bridget Hyde her Receipt Book August the 19th Anno Domini 1676*. Wellcome MS 2990. Welcome Collection, London, England.

James, Edward W. "Libraries in Colonial Virginia." *The William and Mary Quarterly* 3, no. 1 (1894): 43–45.

Jenner, Mark. "From Conduit Community to Commercial Network? Water in London, 1500–1725." In *Londinopolis: Essays in the Cultural and Social History of Early Modern London c. 1500–c. 1750*, edited by Paul Griffiths and Mark S. R. Jenner, 250–72. Manchester: Manchester University Press, 2000.

Jouanna, Jacques. "Water, Health and Disease in the Hippocratic Treatise Airs, Waters, Places." In *Greek Medicine from Hippocrates to Galen: Selected Papers*, edited by Philip van der Eijk, 155–72. Leiden: Brill, 2012.

Kaplan, Amy. "Manifest Domesticity." *American Literature* 70, no. 3 (1998): 581–606.

Keeler, Mary Freer. *The Long Parliament, 1640–1641: A Biographical Study of Its Members*. Philadelphia: American Philosophical Society, 1954.

"kermes, n." *Oxford English Dictionary*. Accessed July 18, 2023, https://doi.org/10.1093/OED/8141402613.

Kernan, Sarah Peters and Helga Müllneritsch, ed. *Culinary Texts in Context, 1500–1800: Manuscript Recipe Books in Early Modern Europe*. Amsterdam: Amsterdam University Press, 2024.

Kingsbury, Susan Myra, ed. *The Records of the Virginia Company of London*, 4 vols. Washington, DC, 1906–35. https://www.loc.gov/item/06035006/.

Knight, Katherine. "A Precious Medicine: Tradition and Magic in Some Seventeenth-Century Household Remedies." *Folklore* 113, no. 2 (2002): 237–47.

Knott, John. "Sir Walter Raleigh's 'Royal Cordial.'" *Dublin Journal of Medical Science* 121 (1906): 63–70, 131–43.

Kok, Su Mei. "'How Many Arts from Such a Labour Flow': Thomas Middleton and London's New River." *Journal of Medieval and Early Modern Studies* 43, no. 1 (2013): 173–90.

Kowalchuk, Kristine. *Preserving on Paper: Seventeenth-Century Englishwomen's Receipt Books*. Toronto: University of Toronto Press, 2017.

Kupperman, Karen Ordahl. "The Puzzle of the American Climate in the Early Colonial Period." *The American Historical Review* 87, no. 5 (1982): 1262–89.

Labaree, Leonard W., ed. *The Papers of Benjamin Franklin,* Vol. 12, *January 1, through December 31, 1765.* New Haven and London: Yale University Press, 1967.

LaCombe, Michael A. *Political Gastronomy: Food and Authority in the English Atlantic World.* Philadelphia: University of Pennsylvania Press, 2012.

Lamb, Jonathan. *Scurvy: The Disease of Discovery.* Princeton: Princeton University Press, 2017.

Lane, Bridget. *Cookery and Medical Remedy Book.* 1737. Clark MS 2015.002. Clark Memorial Library, Los Angeles, CA.

Laroche, Rebecca. "Minding the Fire: Human-Fire Coagency in Margaret Cavendish's *Matrimonial Trouble* and Seventeenth-Century Recipes." In *In the Kitchen, 1550–1800: Reading English Cooking at Home and Abroad,* edited by Madeline Bassnett and Hillary M. Nunn, 221–42. Amsterdam: Amsterdam University Press, 2022.

Laroche, Rebecca and Jennifer Munroe, eds. *Ecofeminist Approaches to Early Modernity.* New York: Palgrave, 2011.

Laroche, Rebecca, Elaine Leong, Jennifer Munroe, Hillary M. Nunn, Amy L. Tigner, and Lisa Smith. "Becoming Visible: Recipes in the Making." *Early Modern Women* 13, no. 1 (2018): 133–43.

Layfield, Anne. *Manuscript Recipes: A Very Interesting MS. Volume of Medical and Household Recipes.* ca. 1640. CPP MS 10a214. College of Physicians of Philadelphia, Philadelphia, PA.

Le Fèbure, Nicaise. *A Compendious Body of Chemistry.* London, 1662.

Le Fèbure, Nicaise. *A Discourse upon Sr Walter Rawleigh's Great Cordial.* London, 1664.

Lemay, J. A. Leo, ed. *Benjamin Franklin: Writings.* New York: Library of America, 1987.

Leong, Elaine. "Collecting Knowledge for the Family: Recipes, Gender, and Practical Knowledge in the Early Modern English Household." *Centaurus* 55 (2013): 81–103.

Leong, Elaine. *Recipes for Everyday Knowledge.* Chicago: University of Chicago Press, 2018.

Levitin, Dmitri. "'Made Up from Many Experimentall Notions': The Society of Apothecaries, Medical Humanism, and the Rhetoric of Experience in 1630s London." *Journal of the History of Medicine and Allied Sciences* 7, no. 4 (2015): 549–87.

Levy, F. J. "How Information Spread among the Gentry, 1550–1640." *Journal of British Studies* 21, no. 2 (1982): 11–34.

Lind, James. *An Essay on Diseases Incidental to Europeans in Hot Climates.* London, 1768.

Lister, Mary. *Recipe Book Known as "Dame Mary Lister's Household Book."* 1625–35. University of Leeds MS 621. University of Leeds, Leeds, England.

Lo Presti, Roberto. "Shaping the Difference: The Medical Inquiry into the Nature of Places and the Early Birth of Anthropology in the Hippocratic Treatise *Airs Waters Places.*" In *Medicine and Space: Body, Surroundings and Borders in Antiquity and the Middle Ages,* edited by Patricia A. Baker, Han Nijdam, and Karine van't Land, 169–95. Leiden: Brill, 2012.

Lupton, Julia Reinhard. "Thinking with Things." *Postmedieval: A Journal of Medieval Cultural Studies* 3, no. 1 (2012): 63–79.

M. B. *The Ladies Cabinet Enlarged and Opened.* London, 1654.

MacGregor, Arthur. "Medicinal Terra Sigillata: A Historical, Geographical and Typological Review." In *A History of Geology and Medicine,* edited by C. J. Duffin, R. T. J. Moody, and C. Gardner-Thorpe, 113–36. London: London Geological Society, 2013.

McCartney, Martha. *Documentary History of Jamestown Island,* Vol. 3, *Biographies of Owners and Residents.* Jamestown Archaeological Assessment, 1992–96. National Park Service. Williamsburg, VA: Colonial Williamsburg Foundation, 2000.

McIlwaine, H. R. *Minutes of the Council and General Court of Colonial Virginia, 1622–32, 1670–76.* Richmond: The Colonial Press, 1924.

McKenney, Thomas Loraine and James Hall. *The Indian Tribes of North America, with Biographical Sketches and Anecdotes of the Principal Chiefs*. Vol. 3. Edinburgh: John Grant, 1934.

Magnaghi, Russell M. "Sassafras and Its Role in Early America, 1562–1662." *Terra Incognitae* 29, no. 1 (1997): 10–21.

Maillard, Kevin Noble. "The Pocahontas Exception: The Exemption of American Indian Ancestry from Racial Purity Law." *Michigan Journal of Race & Law* 12, no. 2 (2007): 351–86.

Manuscript Cookbook. Eighteenth century. MESDA MS VA.M MFm 5A. Museum of Early Southern Decorative Arts (MESDA) Research Center, Old Salem Museums and Gardens, Winston-Salem, NC.

Markatos, Konstantinos, Demetrios Chytas, Demetrios Korres, Konstantinos Laios, Georgios Androutsos, and Efstathios Chronopoulos. "Charles Estienne (1504–1564): His Life, Work, and Contribution to Anatomy and the First Description of the Canal in the Spinal Cord." *World Neurosurgery* 100 (2017): 186–89.

Markham, Gervase. *Countrey Contentments, or The English Husvvife*. London, 1615.

Markham, Gervase. *The English Husbandman*. London, 1613.

Mather, Cotton. *Angel of Bethesda*, edited by Gordon W. Jones. Barre, VT: American Antiquarian Society, 1972.

Maydom, Katrina Elizabeth. "New World Drugs in England's Early Empire." PhD diss., Cambridge University, 2018.

Mayson, Francis. *A Plat of theise Lordships Videlicet Newebrough, Cockewolde, Owleston, Yearsley*. 1605. North Yorkshire County Council County Records Office.

Mentz, Steve. *At the Bottom of Shakespeare's Ocean*. London: Continuum, 2009.

Miscellany. 1613. Folger MS V.a. 260. Folger Shakespeare Library, Washington, DC.

Moffett, Thomas. *Health's Improvement*. London, 1655.

Monardes, Nicolás. *Ioyfull Newes Out of the New-found Worlde*. Translated by John Frampton. London, 1580.

Moore, Lucy. *Lady Fanshawe's Receipt Book: The Life and Times of a Civil War Heroine*. London: Atlantic, 2017.

Morgan, Philip D. *Slave Counterpoint*. Chapel Hill: University of North Carolina Press, 1998.

Munroe, Jennifer. "Sympoeisis and Early Modern Cooking: Troubling the Boundaries of Human/Nonhuman." In *In the Kitchen, 1550–1800: Reading English Cooking at Home and Abroad*, edited by Madeline Bassnett and Hillary M. Nunn, 29–44. Amsterdam: Amsterdam University Press, 2022.

Munroe, Jennifer, Hillary M. Nunn, Margaret Simon and Lisa Smith. "Reconstructing Recipes, Recovering Losses, Telling Stories." *Early Modern Studies Journal* 8 (2022): 1–22.

Mylander, Jennifer. "Early Modern 'How-To' Books: Impractical Manuals and the Construction of Englishness in the Atlantic World." *Journal for Early Modern Cultural Studies* 9, no. 1 (2009): 123–46.

Nashe, Thomas. *Christs Teares Over Ierusalem*. London, 1613.

"The Negro *Caeser*'s Cure for Poison." *Gentleman's Magazine, and Historical Quarterly* 20 (1750): 342–43.

Nicholl, Charles. *The Creature in the Map: A Journey to El Dorado*. Chicago: University of Chicago Press, 1995.

Nicosia, Marissa. "Slaveholding, Seasoning, and the Circulation of Culinary Knowledge in the Frankland Family Receipt Book." In *American Contact: Objects of Intercultural Encounters and the Boundaries of Book History*, edited by Rhae Lynn Barnes and Glenda Goodman, 142–50. Philadelphia: University of Pennsylvania Press, 2024.

Noble, Louise. "A Mythography of Water: Hydraulic Engineering and the Imagination." In *The Palgrave Handbook of Early Modern Literature and Science*, edited by Howard Marchitello and Evelyn Tribble, 445–64. London: Palgrave, 2017.

Norton, Marcy. *Sacred Gifts, Profane Pleasures: A History of Tobacco and Chocolate in the Atlantic World.* Ithaca: Cornell University Press, 2008.

Nunn, Hillary and Rebecca Laroche. "Exploring Manuscripts 10a214." *The Recipes Project*, September 19, 2019. Accessed October 14, 2024. https://recipes.hypotheses.org/thematic-series/exploring-manuscript-10a214.

Nunn, Hillary and Melissa Schultheis. "Using the Methods of Our Manuscripts." Conference Paper, *Modern Language Association Conference*, New York City, NY, January 2018.

Park, Jennifer. "Discandying Cleopatra: Preserving Cleopatra's Infinite Variety in Shakespeare's *Antony and Cleopatra*." *Studies in Philology* 113, no. 3 (2016): 595–633.

Park, Jennifer. "Teaching Recipes, Race, and Erasure in the Early Modern Classroom." *Studies in Medieval and Renaissance Teaching* 28, no. 2 (2021): 61–79.

Parkinson, John. *Paradisi in Sole Paradisus Terrestris. or A Garden of All Sorts of Pleasant Flowers which our English Ayre will Permitt to be Noursed vp.* London, 1629.

Parkinson, John. *Theatrum botanicum: = The Theater of Plants*. London, 1640.

Paster, Gail Kern. "Leaky Vessels: The Incontinent Women of City Comedy." *Renaissance Drama* 18 (1987): 43–65.

Peacham, Henry. *The Gentlemans Exercise*. London, 1612.

Peck, Linda Levy. *Women of Fortune: Money, Marriage, and Murder in Early Modern England.* Cambridge: Cambridge University Press, 2018.

Pelling, Margaret and Frances White. "BUTLER, William." *Physicians and Irregular Medical Practitioners in London 1550–1640 Database*. London, 2004. *British History Online*. Accessed October 14, 2024. https://www.british-history.ac.uk/no-series/london-physicians/1550-1640/butler-william.

Pelling, Margaret and Frances White. "FRASER, Sir Alexander." *Physicians and Irregular Medical Practitioners in London 1550–1640 Database*. London, 2004. *British History Online*. Accessed October 14, 2024. https://www.british-history.ac.uk/no-series/london-physicians/1550-1640/fraser-sir-alexander.

Pelling, Margaret and Frances White. "SHEAF, Thomas." *Physicians and Irregular Medical Practitioners in London 1550–1640 Database*. London, 2004. *British History Online*. Accessed October 14, 2024. https://www.british-history.ac.uk/no-series/london-physicians/1550-1640/sheaf-thomas.

Pencak, William. "Politics and Ideology in *Poor Richard's Almanack*." *The Pennsylvania Magazine of History & Biography* 116, no. 2 (1992): 183–211.

Pennell, Sara. "Perfecting Practice?: Women Manuscript Recipes and Knowledge in Early Modern England." In *Early Modern Women's Manuscript Writing: Selected Papers from the Trinity/Trent Colloquium*, edited by Victoria E. Burke and Jonathan Gibson, 237–58. Basingstoke: Ashgate, 2004.

Pennell, Sara. "Recipes and Reception: Tracking 'New World' Foodstuffs in Early Modern British Culinary Texts, c. 1650–1750." *Food & History* 7 (2009): 11–33.

Pennell, Sara and Michelle DiMeo. "Introduction." In *Reading and Writing Recipe Books, 1500–1800*, edited by Michelle DiMeo and Sara Pennell, 1–22. Manchester: Manchester University Press, 2013.

Percy, George. "Observations by Master George Percy, 1607." In *Narratives of Early Virginia, 1606–1625*, edited by Lyon Gardiner Tyler, 1–23. New York: Scribner's, 1907.

Percy, George. "A Trewe Relacyon of the Procedeinges and Occurrentes of Moment which have hapned in Virginia." *Tyler's Quarterly Magazine* 3 (1922): 260–82.

"Perdita Woman: Lady Elizabeth Ashburnham (later Richardson)." *Perdita Project*. Accessed September 9, 2019.

Philiatros. *Natura Exenterata or, Nature Unbowelled.* London, 1655.

Pinckney, Eliza. *Eliza Pinckney Receipt Book.* 1756. South Carolina Historical Society MS 43-2178. Lowcountry Digital Library, Charleston, SC. Accessed October 14, 2024. https://lcdl.library.cofc.edu/lcdl/catalog/lcdl:51509.

Plat, Hugh. *Delightes for Ladies.* London, 1602.

Pollock, Linda. *With Faith and Physic: The Life of a Tudor Gentlewoman, Lady Grace Mildmay, 1552–1620.* New York: St. Martin's, 1995.

Porter, Roy and G. S. Rousseau. *Gout: The Patrician Malady.* New Haven: Yale University Press, 1998.

Potter, Jennifer. *The Jamestown Brides: The Story of England's Maids for Virginia.* Oxford: Oxford University Press, 2019.

Powell, William S. "Books in the Virginia Colony before 1624." *The William and Mary Quarterly* 5, no. 2 (1948): 177–84.

Price, Lori Lyn. "Gender and Domestic Medicine: Analysis of a Seventeenth-Century Receipt Book." Master's thesis, Harvard Extension School, 2016.

The Queens Closet Opened. London, 1659.

Quinn, David B. "A List of Books Purchased for the Virginia Company." *The Virginia Magazine of History and Biography* 77, no. 3 (1969): 347–60.

Rabb, Theodore K. "'My Lady Sandys her Receipts': A Manuscript of Cookery and Medicine." *The Princeton University Library Chronicle* 72, no. 2 (2011): 454–63.

Rabb, Theodore K. "Sandys, Sir Edwin (1561–1629), Politician and Colonial Entrepreneur." *Oxford Dictionary of National Biography.* September 23, 2004. Accessed July 18, 2023. doi-org.ezproxy.uakron.edu:2443/10.1093/ref:odnb/24650.

Radburn, Nicholas. "'[M]anaged at First as if They Were Beasts': The Seasoning of Enslaved Africans in Eighteenth-Century Jamaica." *Journal of Global Slavery* 6, no. 1 (2021): 11–30.

Raleigh, Walter. *Chemical Recipes.* Late sixteenth century–early seventeenth century. Sloane MS 359. British Library, London, England.

Randolph, Mary. *The Virginia Housewife.* Washington, DC: Davis and Force, 1824.

Rankin, Alisha. "New World Drugs and the Archive of Practice: Translating Nicolás Monardes in Early Modern Europe." *Osiris* 37 (2022): 68–88.

Ransome, David R. "Wives for Virginia, 1621." *The William and Mary Quarterly* 48, no. 1 (1991): 3–18.

The Rates of Merchandizes. That is to Say, the Subsidy of Tonnage, the Subsidy of Poundage, and the Subsidy of Woollen, Cloths or Old Drapery. London, 1642.

The Rates of Marchandizes as they are Set Downe in the Book of Rates. London, 1635.

Rawcliffe, Carole. *Urban Bodies: Communal Health in Late Medieval and English Towns and Cities.* Woodbridge, Suffolk: Boydell, 2013.

Rawdon, Marmaduke. *Medical Receipts.* 1637. University of Minnesota MS WZ250 M489. Owen H. Wangensteen Historical Library of Biology and Medicine, Minneapolis, MN.

Recipe Book. 1663. University of Pennsylvania Ms. Codex 252. University of Pennsylvania, Philadelphia, PA.

Recipe Book. 1765. University of Pennsylvania Ms. Codex 1038. University of Pennsylvania, Philadelphia, PA.

"rheumatoid arthritis, n." *Oxford English Dictionary.* Accessed July 18, 2023, https://doi.org/10.1093/OED/2107230067.

Rivière, Lazare. *The Practice of Physick.* Translated by Nicholas Culpeper, Abdiah Cole and William Rowland. London, 1655.

Robinson, Martha K. "New Worlds, New Medicines: Indian Remedies and English Medicine in Early America." *Early American Studies: An Interdisciplinary Journal* 3, no. 1 (2005): 94–110.

Roebuck, Graham. "Sassafras." In *The Mysterious and the Foreign in Early Modern England*, edited by Helen Ostovich and Mary V. Silcox, 170–86. Newark: University of Delaware Press, 2008.

Rome, Alan S. *The English Embrace of the American Indians: Ideas of Humanity in Early America*. New York: Palgrave, 2017.

Rose, Mary Beth. *Gender and Heroism in Early Modern English Literature*. Chicago: University of Chicago Press, 2002.

Rosenberg, Charles E. "Epilogue: *Airs, Waters, Places*. A Status Report." *Bulletin of the History of Medicine* 86 (2012): 661–70.

Rosvally, Danielle. "Sifting and Sorting: An Introduction to Database Methods and Pedagogy using Humanist Texts." *Early Modern Studies Journal* 9 (2019). https://earlymodernstudiesjournal.org/review_articles/sifting-and-sorting-an-introduction-to-database-methods-and-pedagogy-using-humanist-texts/.

"running water, n." *Oxford English Dictionary*. Accessed September 23, 2023, https://doi.org/10.1093/OED/1111203476.

Rush, Benjamin. *An Oration, delivered February 4, 1774, before the American Philosophical Society, held at Philadelphia*. Philadelphia, 1774.

Saffin-Ellis Miscellany. 1716–62. University of Pennsylvania Ms. Codex 230. University of Pennsylvania, Philadelphia, PA.

St. John, Johanna. *Johanna St. John her Book*. 1680. Wellcome MS 4338. Wellcome Collection, London, England.

Sanderson, Jonathan. "Nicholas Culpeper and the Book Trade: Print and the Promotion of Vernacular Medical Knowledge, 1649–65." PhD diss., University of Leeds, 1999.

Sarkar, Debipriya. *Possible Knowledge: The Literary Forms of Early Modern Science*. Philadelphia: University of Pennsylvania Press, 2023.

Saunders, Richard. *Poor Richard Improved*. Philadelphia, 1768.

Schiebinger, Londa. *Plants and Empire: Colonial Bioprospecting in the Atlantic World*. Boston: Harvard University Press, 2007.

Schiebinger, Londa. *Secret Cures of Slaves: People, Plants, and Medicine in the Eighteenth-Century Atlantic World*. Stanford: Stanford University Press, 2017.

Schmidt, Stephen and Szilvia Szmuk-Tanenbaum. "Manuscript Cookbooks Survey," Project of the Pine Needles Foundation of New York. Accessed October 15, 2024. https://www.manuscriptcookbookssurvey.org.

Schultheis, Melissa. "A Culinary Embassy: Diplomatic Home Making in Lady Ann Fanshawe's *Booke of Receipts*." In *In the Kitchen, 1550–1800: Reading English Cooking at Home and Abroad*, edited by Madeline Bassnett and Hillary M. Nunn, 197–218. Amsterdam: Amsterdam University Press, 2022.

Scott, David. "Constable, Sir William, baronet (bap. 1590, d. 1655), Parliamentarian army officer and Regicide." *Oxford Dictionary of National Biography*. September 23, 2004. Accessed August 28, 2023. doi-org.ezproxy.uakron.edu:2443/10.1093/ref:odnb/6113.

Seelig, Sharon Cadman. *Autobiography and Gender in Early Modern Literature: Reading Women's Lives, 1600–1680*. Cambridge University Press, 2006.

Seth, Suman. *Difference and Disease: Medicine, Race, and the Eighteenth-Century British Empire*. Cambridge: Cambridge University Press, 2018.

Seth, Suman. "Race, Seasoning, and Strangeness: The Problem of Mobility in Early Modern Science and Medicine." *Global Intellectual History* 8, no. 4 (2022): 448–66.

"setwall, n." *Oxford English Dictionary*. Accessed September 2023, https://doi.org/10.1093/OED/4115342106.

Sh., Jo. *A Funeral Elegy on the Right Honourable the Lady Viscountesse Castleton*. London, 1667.

Shahani, Gitanjali G. *Tasting Difference: Food, Race, and Cultural Encounters in Early Modern Literature*. Ithaca: Cornell University Press, 2020.

Shirley, John William. "The Scientific Experiments of Sir Walter Ralegh, the Wizard Earl, and the Three Magi in the Tower 1603–1617." *Ambix* 4, no. 1–2 (1949): 52–66.

Sklar, Kathryn Kish. "Reconsidering Domesticity through the Lens of Empire and Settler Society in North America." *American Historical Review* 124, no. 4 (2019): 1249–66.

Smith, John. *The Generall Historie of Virginia*. London, 1624.

Smith, John. *A Map of Virginia*. London, 1612.

Smith, Geoffrey. "Surviving the Cavalier Winter: The Experience of Richard and Ann Fanshawe." *Parergon* 32, no. 3 (2015): 99–121.

Smith, Geoffrey Ridsill. *In Well Beware: The Story of Newburgh Priory and the Belasyse Family, 1145–1977*. Kineton: Roundwood Press, 1978.

Smith, Lisa. "Medicinal Compounds, Efficacious in Every Case." *The Recipes Project*, January 30, 2013. https://recipes.hypotheses.org/800.

Smith, Pamela H. "Nodes of Convergence, Material Complexes, and Entangled Itineraries." In *Entangled Itineraries: Materials, Practices, and Knowledges across Eurasia*, edited by Pamela H. Smith, 5–24. Pittsburgh: University of Pittsburgh Press, 2019.

Smith, Sean Morey. "Seasoning and Abolition: Humoural Medicine in the Eighteenth-Century British Atlantic." *Slavery & Abolition* 36, no. 4 (2015): 684–703.

Snook, Edith. "English Women's Writing and Indigenous Medical Knowledge in the Early Modern Atlantic World." In *A History of Early Modern Women's Writing*, edited by Patricia Phillippy, 382–97. Cambridge: Cambridge University Press, 2018.

Snook, Edith. "Grace Mildmay's Recipes and Indigenous Knowledge in the Early Modern Atlantic World." *Atlantic Studies* 19, no. 2 (2022): 224–54.

Snook, Edith. "The Recipes of Jonathan Odell and 18th-Century Settler Colonialism in the Maritimes." *Acadiensis* 49, no. 2 (2020): 119–32.

Sorensen, Leni. "Keeping a Good House." *Gastronomica* 5, no. 4 (2005): 106–8.

"spetch, n." *Oxford English Dictionary*. Accessed July 18, 2023, https://doi.org/10.1093/OED/5232610181.

Spiller, Elizabeth. *Seventeenth-Century English Recipe Books: Cooking, Physic and Chirurgery in the Works of Elizabeth Talbot Grey and Aletheia Talbot Howard*. Burlington: Ashgate, 2011.

Stanard, Mary Newton. *The Story of Virginia's First Century*. Philadelphia: Lippincott, 1928.

Stell, P. M. "The Apothecaries of Medieval York." *York Historian* 14 (1976): 26–31.

Stobart, Anne. *Household Medicine in Seventeenth-Century England*. London: Bloomsbury, 2016.

Stobart, Jon. *Sugar and Spice: Grocers and Groceries in Provincial England, 1650–1830*. Oxford: Oxford University Press, 2013.

Sydenham, Thomas. *The Compleat Method of Curing Almost All Diseases*. London, 1694.

Tannenbaum, Rebecca J. *The Healer's Calling: Women and Medicine in Early New England*. Ithaca: Cornell University Press, 2002.

Taylor, John. *Stripping, Whipping, and Pumping, or the Five Mad Shavers of Drury Lane*. London, 1638.

Test, Edward McLean. *Sacred Seeds: New World Plants in Early Modern English Literature*. Lincoln: University of Nebraska Press, 2019.

Tigner, Amy L. "Cake: An Early Modern Chronicle of Trade, Technology, and Exchange." In *In the Kitchen, 1550–1800: Reading English Cooking at Home and Abroad*, edited by Madeline Bassnett and Hillary M. Nunn, 109–30. Amsterdam: Amsterdam University Press, 2022.

Tigner, Amy L. "Trans-border Kitchens: Iberian Recipes in Seventeenth-Century English Manuscripts." *History of Retailing and Consumption* 5, no. 1 (2019): 51–70.

Tryon, Thomas. *The Good House-wife Made a Doctor.* London, 1692.

Tuana, Nancy. "Viscous Porosity: Witnessing Katrina." In *Material Feminisms*, edited by Stacy Alaimo and Susan Hekman, 188–213. Bloomington: Indiana University Press, 2008.

Tyler, Lyon Gardiner. *Encyclopedia of Virginia Biography.* Vol. 1. New York: Lewis Historical Publishing, 1915.

Venieri, Danae, Iosifina Gounaki, George E. Christidis, Charles W. Knapp, Petros Bouras-Vallianatos and Effie Photos-Jones. "Bridging the Gaps: Bole and Terra Sigillata as Artefacts, as Simples and as Antibacterial Clays." *Minerals* 10 (2020): 1–11.

Venner, Tobias. *Via Recta ad Vitam Longam.* London, 1620.

Veracini, Lorenzo. "Introduction: Settler Colonialism as a Distinct Mode of Domination." In *The Routledge Handbook of the History of Settler Colonialism*, edited by Edward Cavanagh and Lorenzo Veracini, 1–8. New York: Routledge, 2016.

Vogel, Virgil J. *American Indian Medicine.* Norman: University of Oklahoma Press, 1970.

Wakeman, Rob. "The Power of the Pot: Naturalizing Carp Through the Early Modern English Receipt Book." In *In the Kitchen, 1550–1800: Reading English Cooking at Home and Abroad*, edited by Madeline Bassnett and Hillary M. Nunn, 131–48. Amsterdam: Amsterdam University Press, 2022.

Walden, Sarah. *Tasteful Domesticity: Women's Rhetoric and the American Cookbook, 1790–1940.* Pittsburgh: University of Pittsburgh Press, 2018.

Walker, Katherine. "Instinct and the Body of the Early Modern Cook." In *In the Kitchen, 1550–1800: Reading English Cooking at Home and Abroad*, edited by Madeline Bassnett and Hillary M. Nunn, 71–88. Amsterdam: Amsterdam University Press, 2022.

Wall, Wendy. "Distillation: Transformations in and out of the Kitchen." In *Renaissance Food from Rabelais to Shakespeare: Culinary Readings and Culinary Histories*, edited by Joan Fitzpatrick, 89–104. Burlington: Ashgate, 2010.

Wall, Wendy. *Recipes For Thought: Knowledge and Taste in the Early Modern Kitchen.* Philadelphia: University of Pennsylvania Press, 2015.

Wall, Wendy. *Staging Domesticity: Household Work and English Identity in Early Modern Drama.* Cambridge: Cambridge University Press, 2002.

Wallis, Patrick. "Apothecaries and the Consumption and Retailing of Medicines in Early Modern London." In *From Physick to Pharmacology: Five Hundred Years of British Drug Retailing*, edited by Louise Hill Curth, 13–28. London: Routledge, 2016.

Wallis, Patrick. "Exotic Drugs and English Medicine: England's Drug Trade, c. 1550–c. 1800." *Social History of Medicine* 25, no. 1 (2012): 20–46.

Wallis, Patrick. "William Bullein." *Oxford Dictionary of National Biography.* Oxford University Press. September 23, 2004. Accessed September 9, 2019. doi-org.ezproxy.uakron.edu:2443/10.1093/ref:odnb/3910.

Watson, Paula and Paul Gauci. "George, 5th Visct. Castleton [I] (1631–1714), of Sandbeck, Yorks." In *The History of Parliament: The House of Commons 1690–1715*, edited by D. Hayton, E. Cruickshanks, and S. Handley. London: Boydell and Brewer, 2002. Accessed October 14, 2024. https://www.historyofparliamentonline.org/volume/1690-1715/member/saunderson-george-1631-1714.

Wear, Andrew. "Place, Health, and Disease: The *Airs, Waters, Places* Tradition in Early Modern England and North America." *Journal of Medieval and Early Modern Studies* 38, no. 3 (2008): 443–65.

Wear, Andrew. "The Prospective Colonist and Strange Environments: Advice on Health and Prosperity." In *Cultivating the Colonies: Colonial States and Their Environmental Legacies*, edited by Christina Folke Ax, et al., 19–46. Athens, OH: Ohio University Press, 2011.

Weatherwise, Abraham. *Father Abraham's Almanack, for the Year of our Lord, 1769.* Philadelphia, 1768.

Weddell, G., ed. *Arcana Fairfaxiana Manuscripta*. Newcastle upon Tyne, 1890.

Welde, Thomas. "Thomas Welde to His Former Parishioners at Tarling, June/July 1632." In *Letters from New England: The Massachusetts Bay Colony 1629–1638*, edited by Everett Emerson, 994–98. Amherst: University of Massachusetts Press, 1976.

White, Susan Reynolds, Sjaak van der Geest, and Anita Hardon. *The Social Lives of Medicine*. Cambridge: Cambridge University Press, 2002.

Wilkins, Sarah Creighton. "For the Rheumatism." *Early Modern Maritime Recipes*. Accessed October 10, 2024. https://emmr.lib.unb.ca/recipes/rheumatism.

Willard, Thomas. "Testing the Waters: Early Modern Studies." In *Bodily and Spiritual Hygiene in Medieval and Early Modern Literature: Explorations of Textual Presentations of Filth and Water*, edited by Albrecht Classen, 568–94. Berlin: De Gruyter, 2017.

Williamson, George C. *Lady Anne Clifford Countess of Dorset, Pembroke & Montgomery*. London: Titus Wilson and Son, 1922.

Willis, Thomas. *The London Practice of Physick*. London, 1684.

Wilson, M. F. *Coxwold parish register transcripts 1583–1666*. Accessed February 3, 2021. https://archive.org/details/CoxwoldParishRegisterTranscripts1583-1666.

Winchcombe, Rachel. *Encountering Early America*. Manchester: Manchester University Press, 2021.

Winche, Rebeckah. *Receipt Book of Rebeckah Winche*. ca. 1666. Folger MS V.b.366. Folger Shakespeare Library, Washington, DC.

Winterbottom, Anna E. "Of the China Root: A Case Study of the Early Modern Circulation of Materia Medica." *Social History of Medicine* 28, no. 1 (2014): 22–44.

Wolfe, Patrick. *Settler Colonialism and the Transformation of Anthropology: The Politics and Poetics of an Ethnological Event*. London: Cassell, 1999.

Woolley, Hannah. *The Accomplish'd Lady's Delight*. London, 1675.

Woolley, Hannah. *The Gentlewomans Companion*. London, 1673.

Working, Lauren. "Pocahontas (c.1595–1617)." In *Lives in Transit in Early Modern England: Identity and Belonging*, edited by Nandini Das, 185–92. Amsterdam: Amsterdam University Press, 2022.

Working, Lauren. "Tobacco and the Social Life of Conquest in London, 1580–1625." *The Historical Journal* 65 (2022): 30–48.

Worshipful Society of the Apothecaries of London. *Medical miscellany* [manuscript]. ca. 1634. Folger MS E.a.5. Folger Shakespeare Library, Washington, DC.

Yates, Julian. *Error, Misuse, Failure*. Minneapolis: University of Minnesota Press, 2003.

Ziser, Michael. "Sovereign Remedies: Natural Authority and the *Counterblaste to Tobacco*." *William and Mary Quarterly* 62, no. 4 (2005): 719–44.

Index